PEDIATRIC COLLEC'

Enriching Pediatric Learning: A Guidebook for Preceptors

EDITOR:

Susan L Bannister, MD, MEd, FRCPC
Editorial Board, *Pediatrics*
Professor, Department of Pediatrics
Cumming School of Medicine, University of Calgary

COMMENTARIES BY:

Robert A Dudas, MD
Associate Professor, Department of Pediatrics
Johns Hopkins University School of Medicine

Karen L Forbes, MD, MEd, FRCPC
Associate Professor, Department of Pediatrics
Faculty of Medicine & Dentistry, University of Alberta

Janice L Hanson, PhD, EdS, MH
Professor of Medicine, Department of Pediatrics
Washington University in St. Louis

Terry Kind, MD, MPH
Professor, Department of Pediatrics
The George Washington University School of Medicine and Health Sciences

Christopher G Maloney, MD, PhD
Professor, Department of Pediatrics
University of Nebraska College of Medicine

Michael S Ryan, MD, MEHP
Associate Professor, Department of Pediatrics
Virginia Commonwealth University School of Medicine

Sandra M Sanguino, MD, MPH
Associate Professor of Pediatrics and Medical Education, Department of Pediatrics
Northwestern University Feinberg School of Medicine

American Academy of Pediatrics

DEDICATED TO THE HEALTH OF ALL CHILDREN®

Published by the
American Academy of Pediatrics
345 Park Blvd.
Itasca, IL 60143

The American Academy of Pediatrics is not responsible for the content of the resources mentioned in this publication. Web site addresses are as current as possible but may change at any time.

Products are mentioned for information purposes only. Inclusion in this publication does not imply endorsement by the American Academy of Pediatrics.

APC025

Print ISBN: 978-1-61002-582-9
eBook ISBN: 978-1-61002-583-6

PEDIATRIC COLLECTIONS

Enriching Pediatric Learning: A Guidebook for Preceptors

Table of Contents

Enriching Pediatric Learning: A Guidebook for Preceptors

About AAP Pediatric Collections

Pediatric Collections is a series of selected pediatric articles that highlight different facets of information across various AAP publications, including AAP Journals, AAP News, Blog Articles, and eBooks. Each series of collections focuses on specific topics in the field of pediatrics so that you can keep up with best practices, and make an informed response to public health matters, trending news, and current events. Each collection includes previously published content focusing on specific topics and articles selected by AAP editors.

Visit http://collections.aap.org to view a list of upcoming collections.

Enriching Pediatric Learning: A Guidebook for Preceptors

Introduction

Medical Education Matters: Pediatric Clinical Teachers Can Inspire the Next Generation of Doctors

By Susan L Bannister, MD, MEd, FRPC

Editorial Board, *Pediatrics*; Professor, Department of Pediatrics, Cumming School of Medicine, University of Calgary

COMSEP, the Council of Medical Student Education in Pediatrics, is a community of pediatric educators committed to supporting each other and delivering excellent pediatric education to medical students. The articles and commentaries in this latest entry in the American Academy of Pediatrics' Pediatric Collections series, entitled *Enriching Pediatric Learning: A Guidebook for Preceptors*, have been written by COMSEP members, and the principles of our organization have driven much of their work.

COMSEP's guiding principles articulate what its members believe to exemplify excellence in medical student education: *Teaching should be excellent, innovative, and scholarly; The learning environment should be safe and enjoyable for all;* and *Patient/family centeredness, teamwork, professionalism, humanism, and service are essential core values of pediatrics.*

Another principle is that *Pediatric medical student education makes all students better doctors.* We recognize that not everyone whom we teach will become a pediatrician, nor will they ultimately care for children in their practice. But we also recognize that many of the skills they learn and the behaviors they observe while working with children, families, and pediatric professionals will influence their growth and may ultimately affect the physicians and surgeons they become. They will learn, for instance, a flexible approach to the physical examination, the power of observation, a way to communicate with 2 very different people at the same time, and the value of communication and teamwork and empathy.

Students recognize this. Several years ago, I asked my students to write down what they learned on their pediatric clerkship that they might apply to other areas of medicine. Here are a few of the things they had to say:

"How to involve families in discussions."

"Sick versus not-sick."

"For adults, similarly evaluating social support networks and home life like we do in kids."

"Empathy for families and parents of kids with chronic diseases."

"Seeing the patient as a whole person in context of family and community."

"Communicating with children and their families."

"Talking with nurses."

"More than anything, compassion for families, patience in medicine."

These students recognize the value of learning in the pediatric clinical environment and can envision how this will influence their future practice.

I often imagine the future interaction of a patient and a medical student. The patient might not even be born yet. The medical student might be in first or second year right now. But they will meet when that medical student does their pediatric clerkship. And when they do, I hope their interaction is based on empathy and teamwork and humanism. And I hope that meeting will influence the future physician the medical student will become. And I believe our work in education, administration, and leadership will play a role in that meeting. And I believe your work as a clinical teacher and the articles in this Pediatric Collection can play a role in that meeting as well.

The 35 articles in this Pediatric Collection have been grouped by themes, and together they describe skills and strategies to improve clinical teaching. The authors and editorial board have tried to imagine the clinical practice of a busy preceptor in a variety of settings—rural or regional or urban practice, community hospital, academic centre—and have tried to provide an article that is succinct and captivating, with practical tips that can be put into use that day with a trainee. We hope this collection, too, will be a practical resource that will support preceptors and educators in their quest to teach, assess, and inspire the medical students with whom they work.

PEDIATRICS PERSPECTIVES

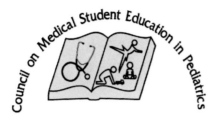

CONTRIBUTORS: Susan L. Bannister, MD,[a] William V. Raszka Jr, MD,[b] and Christopher G. Maloney, MD, PhD,[c]

[a]Department of Pediatrics, University of Calgary, Faculty of Medicine, Calgary, Alberta, Canada; [b]Department of Pediatrics, University of Vermont College of Medicine, Burlington, Vermont; and [c]University of Utah, Department of Pediatrics, Salt Lake City, Utah

Address correspondence to William V. Raszka Jr, MD, Department of Pediatrics, University of Vermont College of Medicine, Given Courtyard, Burlington, VT 05405. E-mail: william.raszka@uvm.edu

Accepted for publication Mar 1, 2010

ABBREVIATION

COMSEP—Council on Medical Student Education in Pediatrics

doi:10.1542/peds.2010-0628

What Makes a Great Clinical Teacher in Pediatrics? Lessons Learned From the Literature

Medical student education in pediatrics has changed significantly over the past 2 decades. There has been an increased emphasis on ambulatory experiences and greater use of community- and ambulatory-based faculty.[1,2] A shift from inpatient to more outpatient primary care and subspecialty rotation experiences combined with productivity and academic demands may result in faculty spending less time with students.[3] However, these same faculty, often with little formal training, are critical to the pediatric education of medical students. The goal of this article is to review the peer-reviewed literature that describes the attributes and skills of a great clinical teacher, whether community or university based, and outline some strategies used to enhance medical student learning.

TEACHING IN THE CLINICAL SETTING First, what is a clinical teacher? The Council on Medical Student Education in Pediatrics (COMSEP) defines a clinical teacher as someone who interacts with a student in the context of ongoing patient care. The feature that sets clinical teachers apart from other types of teachers, then, is the involvement of, and teaching about, a patient. Teaching in the clinical setting is complicated, because the preceptor needs not only to diagnose and treat the patient but also the student. The preceptor needs to learn what knowledge or skills the student does or does not have and ensure that the student has progressed to where he or she needs to be by the end of the session. The educational goal of clinical teachers, and a primary goal of our work in COMSEP, is to ensure that students are prepared to practice effective patient-centered care.

ATTRIBUTES OF A GREAT CLINICAL TEACHER We can all remember during medical school or residency having teachers that made the experience memorable and inspired us to work a little harder, study a little longer, and sleep a little less. Unfortunately, we can also remember teachers who made the learning experience either unsatisfying or at least less enjoyable. Distinguishing between these 2 types of teachers is of keen interest to all educators.[4] The results of several studies have suggested that great clinical teachers possess both unique noncognitive and cognitive attributes.[5,6] In a review of the literature on effective clinical teaching published between 1909 and 2006, 480 unique descriptors of good teaching were classified into 49 themes. Although cognitive attributes such as knowledge and procedural skills are important (as shown in Table 1), noncognitive attributes play equally important roles.

Noncognitive Attributes

For example, consider the key role of enthusiasm in a great clinical teacher.[6–8] The importance of enthusiasm is not a new concept. In the 19th century, Ralph Waldo Emerson wrote, "Nothing great was ever accomplished without enthusiasm," and Samuel Taylor Coleridge wrote, "Nothing is so contagious as enthusiasm." Enthusiasm is not necessar-

TABLE 1 Key Cognitive and Noncognitive Attributes of Clinical Teachers as Found in the Literature[5–11,13]

Cognitive	Noncognitive
Is knowledgeable	Is enthusiastic
Demonstrates clinical skills	Is stimulating
Is well organized	Is encouraging
Has excellent communication skills	Creates a positive, supportive learning environment
Provides feedback	Models professional characteristics
Explains concepts clearly	Focuses on learner's needs
Sets goals and expectations	Interacts positively with students
Provides direct supervision	Listens

ily characterized by boisterousness but by an authentic passion. Passion can be directed to patient care, the education of the student, or, preferably, to both. In the classroom, enthusiastic teachers make eye contact, are animated, and infuse the session with energy. In the context of clinical teaching, enthusiastic teachers are excited by the presence of the medical student and infuse the patient and student interactions with a natural, unforced energy. Enthusiastic teachers capture students' attention, excite them about learning the practice of medicine, and, by stimulating reflection, promote student learning.[9]

Although a great number of noncognitive attributes other than enthusiasm are highly valued, most can be summarized by a single word: respect. As Ralph Waldo Emerson also wrote, "the secret of education is respecting the student." A great teacher recognizes that the student-teacher relationship is a bidirectional exchange. We learn from the literature that the great clinical teacher is nonjudgmental, develops a positive relationship with students, creates a supportive learning environment, and listens to what the student has to say.[5,7,8,10] Memorable teachers focus on the learners' needs rather than their own teaching interests and involve the learners in setting relevant educational goals.[11] Students thrive when their opinions and views are valued and they are allowed to voice their views in a safe, supportive environment.

Great clinical teachers also serve as professional role models and mentors for students, which is a complex and purposeful activity that involves not only modeling clinical competence but also professionalism. The clinical teacher occupies the role to which the student aspires. In that role, did the clinical teacher show genuine concern for patients, recognize his or her own limitations, show respect for others, and take responsibility for his or her actions?[9] The student quickly learns whether the observed behaviors are either acceptable or worth emulating. The importance of appropriate role-modeling cannot be underestimated. In a study that looked at medical students at the beginning and midway through their clerkship year, observation and par-

ticipation in unprofessional behaviors increased and students increasingly perceived unprofessional behaviors as being appropriate.[12]

Cognitive Attributes

When faculty and residents are individually asked to rank the critical characteristics of clinical teachers, both rank clinical competence as the most important cognitive quality.[7,8] Great clinical teachers are universally expected to be not only clinically competent but also able to demonstrate and explain clinical skills.[5,7,10] They use highly developed communication skills to converse with patients, families, members of the health care team, and students.[8] Moreover, they articulate their thought processes and describe the clinical patterns used to make clinical decisions with clarity and in language the student understands.[9,13]

The great clinical teacher relies on a variety of skills and strategies to enhance medical student learning. Briefly, great clinical teachers set goals with students and hold them accountable. Students highly value setting goals, debriefing after clinical encounters, being involved with patient management decisions, and receiving timely feedback in a learning environment that combines both independence and supervision.[10] Direct, competent supervision, particularly when combined with focused feedback, positively influences both patient care and student education.[14] In a study of more than 1200 medical students who had completed their clinical rotations, supervision correlated far better with the overall effectiveness of the clinical rotation than patient mix and numbers of patients seen.[15]

SUMMARY Great clinical teachers occupy a unique and powerful role in the education of medical students. Their noncognitive and cognitive actions and behaviors influence future student behaviors and career choices and, most importantly, result in a future generation of physicians who are equipped to care for children.[16] Although we continue to have difficulty defining the critical characteristics of a great clinical teacher, identifying such a teacher is easy: they are the ones to whom students and residents flock. If we return to a teacher we each remember as having made the clinical experience memorable and inspired us to work a little harder, it is the person, not necessarily the content, that we remember. Although some have advocated that great teaching is innate,[13] many of the skills and strategies can, in fact, be learned and developed. Over the next several issues we will explore in greater detail the skills and strategies developed by COMSEP that can be quickly and efficiently assimilated into daily practice and help make a good clinical teacher great.

REFERENCES

1. White CB, Waller JL, Freed G, et al. The state of undergraduate pediatric medical education in North America: the COMSEP survey. *Teach Learn Med.* 2007;19(3):264–270

2. Fields SA, Usatine R, Steiner E. Teaching medical students in the ambulatory setting: strategies for success. *JAMA.* 2000;283(18):2362–2364

3. Mooradian AD, Meenrajan S. The business of academic medicine is a business like no other: a perspective. *Health Care Manag (Frederick).* 2009;28(4):344–350

4. Ripley A. What makes a great teacher? Available at: www.theatlantic.com/magazine/archive/2010/01/what-makes-a-great-teacher/7841. Accessed February 26, 2010

5. Irby DM. Teaching and learning in ambulatory care settings: a thematic review of the literature. *Acad Med.* 1995;70(10):898–931

6. Sutkin G, Wagner E, Harris I, Schiffer R. What makes a good clinical teacher in medicine? A review of the literature. *Acad Med.* 2008;83(5):452–466

7. Masunaga H, Hitchcock MA. Residents' and faculty's beliefs about the ideal clinical teacher. *Fam Med.* 2010;42(2):116–120

8. Buchel TL, Edwards FD. Characteristics of effective clinical teachers. *Fam Med.* 2005;37(1):30–35

9. Irby DM. Effective clinical teaching & learning: clinical teaching and the clinical teacher. Available at: www.med.cmu.ac.th/secret/meded/ct2.htm. Accessed February 25, 2010

10. Goertzen J, Stewart M, Weston W. Effective teaching behaviours of rural family medicine preceptors. *CMAJ.* 1995;153(2):161–168

11. Menachery EP, Wright SM, Howell EE, Knight AM. Physician-teacher characteristics associated with learner-centered teaching skills. *Med Teach.* 2008;30(5):e137–e144

12. Reddy ST, Farnan JM, Yoon JD, et al. Third-year medical students' participation in and perceptions of unprofessional behaviors. *Acad Med.* 2007;82(10 suppl):S35–S39

13. Gibson J. The five "Es" of an excellent teacher. *Clin Teach.* 2009;6(1):3–8

14. Kilminster SM, Jolly BC. Effective supervision in clinical practice settings: a literature review. *Med Educ.* 2000;34(10):827–840

15. Dolmans DH, Wolfhagen IH, Essed GG, et al. The impacts of supervision, patient mix, and numbers of students on the effectiveness of clinical rotations. *Acad Med.* 2002;77(4):332–335

16. Hauer KE, Durning SJ, Kernan WN, et al. Factors associated with medical students' career choices regarding internal medicine. *JAMA.* 2008;300(10):1154–1164

FINANCIAL DISCLOSURE: *The authors have indicated they have no financial relationships relevant to this article to disclose.*

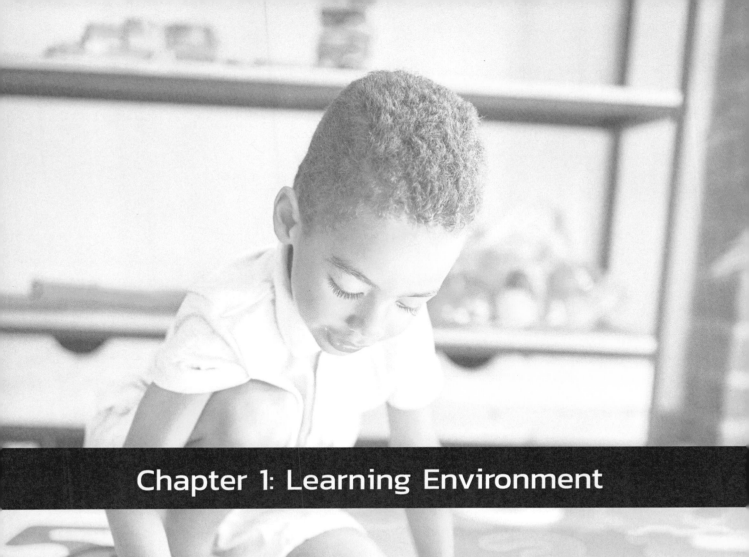

Chapter 1: Learning Environment

Chapter 1

Fostering Humanism in Pediatrics: The Importance of Developing Non-Cognitive Skills in a Supportive Learning Environment

By Michael S Ryan, MD, MEHP
Associate Professor in Pediatrics, Virginia Commonwealth University School of Medicine

Take a moment and consider: Who was the best clinical teacher you had the opportunity to learn from in your career?

Have someone in mind?

If so, consider the attributes that made them so outstanding. Were those attributes related to their knowledge base—or something else?

Chances are, the person in mind inspired you, communicated effectively, supported your development as a learner, and integrated you into patient care activities. They likely possessed a reasonable medical knowledge base, but that may not be what you recall most. A recent literature review has demonstrated exactly that: Possession of outstanding non-cognitive skills is what transforms good clinical teaching to excellent clinical teaching.[1] These interpersonal and humanistic qualities advance the education mission and inspire future generation of physicians.

Over the last half century our profession has developed a profound interest in cultivating the humanistic physician. This desire was a counter-response to the gradual shift toward corporatization of healthcare and de-emphasis of the patient-doctor relationship.[2] As a consequence, the medical education community endorsed a variety of systematic changes. Most notably, the Arnold P. Gold foundation was founded in recognition of its namesake, a pediatric neurologist who practiced medicine with a level of unparalleled humanism and dedication. The foundation formalized the white coat ceremony to recognize the professional responsibility of becoming a physician and established funding to promote and award humanistic behavior among physicians and trainees.[3]

In the present day, at a time when our profession struggles with challenges centered on burnout, mistreatment, disparities, and the larger learning climate,[4] it is perhaps even more important to train clinician-teachers to practice humanistic medicine. Recognition of the value in cultivating the humanistic clinician-teacher is ingrained in the culture of the Council on Medical Student Education in Pediatrics (COMSEP). Two of its early leaders, Rich Sarkin and Steve Miller, practiced and emphasized humanism in medicine and collaboration between learners and teachers.[5] Despite their untimely deaths in 2004, the memory and philosophy of Rich and Steve are continually present in the COMSEP community.

This chapter contains 4 instrumental articles that would make Rich and Steve proud. Collectively, they provide strategies to create a learning environment that fosters learning, humanism, and growth.

Taking the lens of self-determined learning theory, Dudas and Bannister describe the "non-cognitive" attributes of exceptional clinician-educators.[6] They emphasize the importance of not just *what* we teach, but *how* we teach. It is a pediatrician's enthusiasm, role-modeling abilities, willingness to allow students opportunities to practice, and approach to lifelong learning that sets them apart.

In the next paper, the focus is the learning environment.[7] The authors describe the value in setting expectations up front, which includes planning for the arrival of medical students and welcoming them into the environment upon their arrival. Through the emphasis on establishing a conducive learning climate, the environment itself can foster an outstanding relationship between learner and clinician-educator.

Continuing with the learning climate theme, Young and colleagues describe the significant threat posed by microaggressions.[8] Within the clinical setting, microaggressions are comments or actions that often result in an impaired experience for the learner. The authors start by defining the term and then summarize the literature around its pervasiveness. Importantly, a series of opportunities are provided to address this issue. These remedies are offered at the level of the learner-educator, the educator themselves, and finally for institutions and society more globally.

The final paper in this chapter defines and describes methods for bringing humanism into our daily teaching practice.[9] Plant and colleagues outline the value of humanistic practice, both in terms of its application for education and the impact on patient care outcomes. The authors emphasize the humility, intellectual curiosity, and high standards of professional behavior that are common in humanistic physicians. They then provide specific teaching strategies to teach humanism while providing clinical care.

Taken collectively, we anticipate these articles will provide a foundation to one's continued growth as an outstanding and humanistic clinician-teacher.

References

1. Sutkin G, Wagner E, Harris I, Schiffer R. What makes a good clincal teacher in medicine? A review of the literature. *Academic Medicine*. 2008; 83: 452-466.
2. Thibault GE. Humanism in medicine: what does it mean and why is it more important than ever? *Academic Medicine*. 2019; 94: 1074-1077.
3. The Arnold P. Gold Foundation. https://www.gold-foundation.org/about-us/
4. Dyrbye LN, Massie FS Jr, Eacker A, Harper W, Power D, Durning SJ, Thomas MR, Moutier C, Satele D, Sloan J, et al. 2010. Relationship between burnout and professional conduct and attitudes among US medical students. *JAMA*. 304:1173–1180.
5. First, L.R., Greenberg, L., and Siegel, B. In memoriam: a tribute to the lives of Steve Miller and Rich Sarkin. *Ambulatory Pediatrics*. 2005; 5: 1–2.
6. Dudas RA, Bannister SL. It's not just what you know: the non-cognitive attributes of great clinical teachers. *Pediatrics*. 2014; 134: 852-4.
7. Bannister SL, Hanson JL, Maloney CG, Dudas RA. Practical framework for fostering a positive learning environment. *Pediatrics*. 2015; 136: 6-9.
8. Young K, Punnett A, Suleman S. A little hurts a lot: exploring the impact of microaggressions in pediatric medical education. *Pediatrics*. 2020. 146. e20201636.
9. Plant J, Barone MA, Serwint JR, Butani L. Taking humanism back to the bedside. *Pediatrics*. 2015; 136: 828-30.

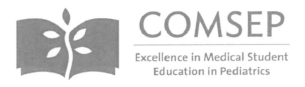

COMSEP

Excellence in Medical Student
Education in Pediatrics

AUTHORS: Robert A. Dudas, MD,[a] and Susan L. Bannister, MD[b]

[a]*Department of Pediatrics, Johns Hopkins University School of Medicine, Baltimore, Maryland; and*[b]*Department of Pediatrics, University of Calgary, Faculty of Medicine, Calgary, Alberta, Canada*

Address correspondence to Robert A. Dudas, MD, Department of Pediatrics, Johns Hopkins Bayview Medical Center, 4940 Eastern Ave, Baltimore, MD 21224. E-mail: rdudas@jhmi.edu

Accepted for publication Jul 29, 2014

Dr Dudas drafted the initial manuscript, conceptualized the ideas presented, coordinated data collection, and reviewed and revised the manuscript; Dr Bannister conceptualized the ideas presented, coordinated data collection, and reviewed and revised the manuscript; and both authors approved the final manuscript as submitted.

KEY WORDS
medical education, teaching

ABBREVIATIONS
COMSEP—Council on Medical Student Education in Pediatrics
SDT—self-determination theory

doi:10.1542/peds.2014-2269

It's Not Just What You Know: The Non-Cognitive Attributes of Great Clinical Teachers

Although it is understood that great clinical teachers are knowledgeable about their subject matter, expertise in a given field does not always translate to excellence in teaching. This article resumes the series by the Council on Medical Student Education in Pediatrics (COMSEP) examining the skills and strategies of great clinical teachers.[1] Great clinical teachers recognize that "how" they teach is just as important as "what" they teach. This "how" consists of 2 parts: a positive learning environment[2] and an enthusiastic, motivating, and respectful teacher.[3,4] In an upcoming article, we will outline the benefits and structure of such a learning environment. But first, drawing from the medical education, business, leadership, and sports literature, we will consider "how" great clinical teachers get the best out of their students. They motivate them, they are enthusiastic, they are both leaders and coaches, they remain students themselves, and they have strategies for when things go wrong.

ENCOURAGE SELF-MOTIVATION

Students will have difficulty mastering a subject if they are not internally motivated to do so.[5] Self-determination theory (SDT) provides a useful framework with which to consider students' motivation. According to this framework, the motivation to learn is driven by 3 psychological needs: a sense of relatedness, a sense of autonomy, and a sense of competence.[6] In the best-selling book *Drive*, Daniel Pink examines how this framework operates and finds that a sense of purpose is also important to achieve optimal performance.[7]

There are multiple ways that clinical teachers can establish an environment in which students are self-motivated to do well (Table 1).

BE ENTHUSIASTIC

> *"Nothing great was ever accomplished without enthusiasm"*
>
> Ralph Waldo Emerson

In almost all the studies of great clinical teachers, enthusiasm emerges as 1 of the most important characteristics.[3,9,10] Enthusiastic teachers are not necessarily boisterous, but rather they are energetic and authentically passionate about both the subject matter and teaching. These teachers are delighted to be at work and even more delighted when a student joins them. And students do (they flock to these teachers and are excited to work alongside them). Enthusiastic teachers use vocal animation by varying their volume (sometimes speaking with a whisper) and their rate of speech (slowing down articulation for emphasis), by repeating words and pausing for emphasis. They smile and gesture, maintain eye contact, nod, and are genuinely thrilled to be teaching.[11]

BE A LEADER

Great leaders and great clinical teachers share several key behaviors. They Model the way, Enable others to act, and Encourage the heart.[12] "Model the way" suggests that great clinical teachers set

TABLE 1 Ways Clinical Teachers Can Establish an Environment to Self-Motivate Students

Psychological Need	General Principle	Specific Action
Relatedness	Treat students collegially	Introduce them to the team and make sure everyone knows each other's names and roles[8]
	Integrate the student into the clinical environment through orientation	Show the student how things work, where and how clinical work is done
		Give the student a place to put their things and a place to work and study
	Value the personal lives of students	Ask about non-medical topics such as outside interests and identify areas of common interest
		Ask about career interests and learning objectives
	Offer emotional support	Periodically "check in" to see how they are faring with the stresses of the clinical environment
	Maximize continuity in the relationship between preceptor and student as well as between student and patient/family	Make efforts to align schedules
		Try to keep patient assignments the same for consecutive days, arrange follow-up of outpatients when the student is back in clinic
	Allow students to build meaningful relationships with patients	Allow students sufficient time with patients/families
		Value these relationships
Autonomy	As much as possible, give students choices	Within reason, let students select which things to do, when to do them, how to do them
		Encourage students to direct discussions based on their learning needs as they become apparent during clinical encounters
	Allow students' plans or ideas to prevail, even if it is not what the teacher would otherwise do	Ask their opinions about patient management
		Use their clinical plans as long as they are safe, evidenced-based care
Competence	Enable students to feel that they know something or are able to do something	Observe students with patients and then match levels of supervision and autonomy with levels of competence
	Allow students to experience mastery	Have students teach: you, each other, families, staff
Purpose	Help students see how what they are doing connects to a larger purpose	"I know you are not going into pediatrics but here is how this applies to being a physician"
		Connect what they are doing with their personal goals

an example as they teach and practice medicine. Excellent teachers are aware that students are constantly watching their behaviors, both good and bad, and they explicitly articulate the thinking behind their actions. They recognize the importance of modeling humanistic behaviors such as empathy, respect, and compassion. They engage in reflective practice, set goals, acknowledge weaknesses, and treat patients and students with the utmost of care and respect. They "walk the talk" by behaving in a manner that is consistent

with what they would say comprises excellent clinical care.

"Enable others to act" stresses collaboration and teamwork, and reminds us of the importance of ensuring that medical students have the skills and resources to do their work well. It means pushing learners into more senior roles along a spectrum of clinical autonomy and providing increasingly challenging tasks to encourage their development as clinicians. Teachers who practice this positively influence medical students through an atmosphere of

trust, mutual respect, and belief in their abilities.[5]

"Encourage the heart" proposes that teachers recognize and value the contributions that medical students make (to patients, to inter- or multidisciplinary teams, to the preceptor him or herself, and to the student's own learning). They believe in the abilities of the learner, offer positive reinforcement, and lend support. It means celebrating accomplishments, both big and small. Many of us can recall the pediatricians who would give each resident a bottle of champagne to celebrate his or her first clear lumbar puncture.

BE A COACH

"Coaching done well may be the most effective intervention designed for human performance."

Gawande A.[13]

Great clinical teachers, like great athletic coaches, know when to push and when to support. Anson Dorrance and Patrick Riley are renowned for their respective dominances in coaching women's college soccer and men's professional basketball.[14,15] They inspired their players to believe anything was possible and then encouraged them to go out on the field or onto the court and achieve it.[14,15] They expected their athletes to stay the course, pursue mastery, overcome setbacks, and fulfill their potential.[14,15] Similarly, clinical teaching strives for these same outcomes. It requires a longitudinal relationship between teacher and student that allows for repetitive practice, ongoing assessment via direct observation, and effective feedback.

Great teachers remember what it felt like to be a medical student (they acknowledge that learning medicine and caring for patients is hard and taxing and, at times, frightening). Like a coach, they help their students focus on "what's important now" when in the midst of challenging clinical circumstances.[16]

BE A STUDENT

"No man can teach successfully who is not at the same time a student."

Sir William Osler

Great clinical teachers are students at heart. They model life-long learning by "looking things up" in a transparent manner; they welcome feedback on their own teaching and clinical performance and engage in deliberate practice.[17] Great clinical teachers strive to improve their own clinical and teaching skills and knowledge. They realize there is much to learn and many to learn from, including their own students.

BE PREPARED FOR WHEN THINGS GO WRONG

Great clinical teachers know that, sometimes, teaching and learning don't work out as expected or hoped. They will attempt to diagnose the learning or teaching challenge by recognizing that there are a multitude of reasons students struggle. They will consider motivation, and determine if a student's difficulties are related to a lack of motivation (won't do) or to a lack of skills and knowledge (can't do).[18] Such teachers then tailor their intervention to either self-motivate learners (see Table 1) or assist learners in acquiring the needed knowledge and skills.

Another framework, adapted from the clinical domain of Family Medicine,[19] encourages a teacher to explore a student's feelings, ideas, impact on function, and expectations about a particular learning challenge. Using this model, a great clinical teacher will work with the learner to establish a common ground[19] to address challenges.

Great clinical teachers are humble and will often seek to find what gap in their own teaching skill has led to struggles for a learner. They will go to colleagues and review learner scenarios with them, "bouncing" these off others to get perspective and guidance.

CONCLUSIONS

Great clinical teachers recognize that "how" they teach is just as important as "what" they teach. They view students as future colleagues and feel privileged to have a role in their education. They teach by being enthusiastic, by self-motivating students, and by being a leader and a coach. And as new technologies provide students with easy and immediate access to medical knowledge, great clinical teachers realize that "how" they teach may be even more important, memorable, and inspiring to students' success than "what" they teach.

REFERENCES

1. Bannister SL, Raszka WV Jr, Maloney CG. What makes a great clinical teacher in pediatrics? Lessons learned from the literature. *Pediatrics*. 2010;125(5):863–865

2. Genn JM. AMEE Medical Education Guide No. 23 (Part 1): Curriculum, environment, climate, quality and change in medical education-a unifying perspective. *Med Teach*. 2001;23(4):337–344

3. Sutkin G, Wagner E, Harris I, Schiffer R. What makes a good clinical teacher in medicine? A review of the literature. *Acad Med*. 2008;83(5):452–466

4. Hatem CJ, Searle NS, Gunderman R, et al. The educational attributes and responsibilities of effective medical educators. *Acad Med*. 2011;86(4):474–480

5. Kusurkar RA, Croiset G, Galindo-Garre F, Ten Cate O. Motivational profiles of medical students: association with study effort, academic performance and exhaustion. *BMC Med Educ*. 2013;13:87. doi: 10.1186/1472-6920-13-87

6. Schumacher DJ, Englander R, Carraccio C. Developing the master learner: applying learning theory to the learner, the teacher, and the learning environment. *Acad Med*. 2013;88(11):1635–1645

7. Pink DH. *Drive: The Surprising Truth About What Motivates Us*. New York, NY: Riverhead Books; 2009

8. Bannister SL, Wickenheiser HM, Keegan DA. Key elements of highly effective teams. *Pediatrics*. 2014;133(2):184–186

9. Buchel TL, Edwards FD. Characteristics of effective clinical teachers. *Fam Med*. 2005;37(1):30–35

10. Masunaga H, Hitchcock MA. Residents' and faculty's beliefs about the ideal clinical teacher. *Fam Med*. 2010;42(2):116–120

11. Tauber R, Mester C. *Acting Lessons For Teachers: Using Performance Skills in the Classroom*. Westport, CT: Praeger; 1994

12. Kouzes J, Posner B. *The Leadership Challenge*, 4th ed. San Francisco, CA: Jossey-Bass; 2007

13. Gawande A. Personal best: top athletes and singers have coaches. Should you? *The New Yorker*. October 3, 2011. Available at: www.newyorker.com/reporting/2011/10/03/111003fa_fact_gawande?currentPage=all. Accessed September 21, 2014

14. Crothers T. *The Man Watching: A Biography of Anson Dorrance, the Unlikely Architect of the Greatest College Sports Dynasty Ever*. New York, NY: Thomas Dunne Books; 2006

15. Riley P. *The Winner Within: A Life Plan for Team Players*. New York, NY: GP Putnam's Sons; 1993

16. Holtz L. *Winning Every Day*. New York, NY: Harper Business; 1998

17. Ericsson KA. Deliberate practice and acquisition of expert performance: a general overview. *Acad Emerg Med*. 2008;15(11):988–994

18. Daniels A. *Bringing Out the Best in People*. New York, NY: McGraw-Hill; 2000

19. Stewart M, Brown J, eds. *Patient Centered Medicine: Transforming the Clinical Method*. Thousand Oaks, CA: Sage Publications; 1995

FINANCIAL DISCLOSURE: The authors have indicated they have no financial relationships relevant to this article to disclose.
FUNDING: No external funding.
POTENTIAL CONFLICT OF INTEREST: The authors have indicated they have no potential conflicts of interest to disclose.

Practical Framework for Fostering a Positive Learning Environment

Susan L. Bannister, MD, MEd[a], Janice L. Hanson, PhD, EdS[b], Christopher G. Maloney, MD, PhD[c], Robert A. Dudas, MD[d]

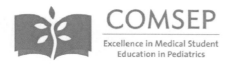

[a]University of Calgary, Faculty of Medicine, Calgary, Alberta, Canada; [b]University of Colorado School of Medicine, Denver, Colorado; [c]University of Utah School of Medicine and Primary Children's Hospital, Salt Lake City, Utah; and [d]Johns Hopkins School of Medicine, Baltimore, Maryland

Dr Bannister conceptualized and drafted the initial manuscript; and all authors reviewed and revised the manuscript and approved the final manuscript as submitted.

www.pediatrics.org/cgi/doi/10.1542/peds.2015-1314

DOI: 10.1542/peds.2015-1314

Accepted for publication Apr 22, 2015

Address correspondence to Susan L. Bannister, Department of Pediatrics, Faculty of Medicine, University of Calgary, 2888 Shaganappi Trail NW, Calgary, Alberta, Canada T3B 6A8. E-mail: susanl.bannister@albertahealthservices.ca

PEDIATRICS (ISSN Numbers: Print, 0031-4005; Online, 1098-4275).

FINANCIAL DISCLOSURE: The authors have indicated they have no financial relationships relevant to this article to disclose.

FUNDING: No external funding was secured for this study.

POTENTIAL CONFLICT OF INTEREST: The authors have indicated they have no potential conflicts of interest to disclose.

The Council on Medical Student Education in Pediatrics continues the series about skills of, and strategies used by great clinical teachers. Great clinical teachers recognize that many things influence students' learning, including what they teach, how they teach, and where they teach.[1,2] "Where" refers to the learning environment. Although the term "environment" may conjure visions of trees, snow-capped mountains, and rain, the "learning environment" refers to the setting in which the curriculum exists. The learning environment includes the physical, social, and psychological context in which students learn and the overall atmosphere or culture pervading the setting where students and clinical teachers work and learn together.[3,4] Although the learning environment of an institution is greatly influenced at the organizational level, this article will focus on elements under the control of individual teachers. We describe practical ways busy clinical teachers can foster a positive learning environment.

WHY A POSITIVE LEARNING ENVIRONMENT IS IMPORTANT

A positive learning environment helps students succeed,[5] affects their moral development,[6] and models a humanistic approach to medicine.[7] Recently, the Association of American Medical Colleges released a statement on the optimal learning environment.[8] However, for decades, great clinical teachers have known that the learning environment affects ethical and personal development.[9] Orienting students leads to improved preparedness for clinical work,[10] and encouraging students to be active participants in the learning process leads to enhanced learning.[11] In addition, the presence of exemplary role models enhances learning.[12]

HOW TO CREATE A POSITIVE LEARNING ENVIRONMENT

Clinical teachers foster a positive learning environment in many practical ways (Table 1). In pediatrics, students worry about "breaking" a child, "dropping a baby," "hurting" a child, not knowing how to relate to children, and not knowing how to examine "such a small baby" or calm a baby down.[13] They also worry about the parents' reactions, dealing with "2 things at once" (the parent and the child), "moms yelling" at them, and not knowing what to say to parents or how to answer their questions.[13]

Teachers have a role in addressing these concerns explicitly, giving students practical tips in communicating with patients and families, and examining patients in developmentally appropriate ways. Ideally, the conversation occurs at the beginning of a teacher-student interaction (whether the start of a shift in the emergency department or the first day of a multiweek experience). Great clinical teachers provide practical tips about working with pediatric patients and families, such as being flexible with the order of the physical exam, adjusting the history and physical exam to the developmental age of the child, using parents as allies in the physical exam, talking to patients about their interests, getting down to the patient's level, and appreciating the

TABLE 1 Practical Ways Clinical Teachers Can Enhance the Learning Environment[5,21–23]

Important Aspects of a Positive Learning Environment	Practical Ways to Make This Happen
Preceptor aware of resources available at course/clerkship and institution level	Have a list of contact names and numbers for student affairs, mental health support, clerkship director, etc.
Students feel expected	Contact students before rotation. Explain where to park, when and where to arrive, how to dress, what to bring.[10]
Students feel welcome	Orient students upon arrival. Give them a place to put their coat, backpack, lunch, etc. Introduce student to nurses, receptionist, and other people in learning environment.[10,14]
Students have a space to learn	Allow students to use your internet, textbooks. Ideally, have a desk or some sort of space for students.
Students have autonomy	Ideally, have students see patients on their own while the preceptor continues to see other patients.
Students are part of learning process	Make sure students are aware of, and contribute to, objectives and learning schedule.
Communication is open	Model open communication with students and all members of the health care team.[14]
Observation occurs	Observe students in a focused, direct way.[17]
Feedback occurs regularly	Provide concrete feedback.[18]
Students have opportunities to show their progress	Provide opportunities to practice after feedback, then observe the targeted skill again, so that students can demonstrate progress.[19]
Questions are asked in a respectful way	Pay attention to how questions are asked. Construct questions based on students' ability.[24]
The environment is respectful	Model respectful communication with students, patients, families, and all members of the health care team.
Students have ample time to learn and participate in other activities (concept of wellness)	Schedule time for students to study on their own as well as time for students to pursue outside interests.
Students feel supported	Inquire as to how students are doing. Direct students to student affairs office, faculty advisor (if applicable), and other resources at medical school if needed.
Students receive assistance in realizing the meaning of learning	Articulate how learning will positively influence students' roles as future physicians.
Students are excited to learn	Create an environment in which students are eager to participate and learn.
Students experience positive peer interactions	Consider teaching 2 students at a time.
Students' roles are clear	Make expectations clear. Make sure students understand their roles and the roles of all members of health care team.[14]

fun and playfulness of this patient population.[13]

We have organized, in a typical timeline, actions great clinical teachers take to create a positive learning environment, from before students arrive to the end of their clinical experience.

BEFORE STUDENTS ARRIVE

Fostering a positive learning environment begins before students arrive to work with a teacher. Although administrative logistics are not a highlight of this article, knowing the course or clerkship director and how to contact him or her with questions or concerns is important. Clarifying the clerkship director's expectations for students in clinical settings and criteria for assessment and grading prepares the teacher to explain these parameters to students when they arrive, so students know from the beginning the basis for assessment in the clinical setting.

Before they arrive, students need to be oriented regarding the location of the clinical experience and expectations such as when to arrive, how to prepare, and what to bring.[10] Students should be made aware if they are supposed to be in different locations on different days (for instance, for school visits, multidisciplinary meetings, or grand rounds). Alerting students about the medical tools they do or do not need to bring allows the student to arrive prepared. Letting students know the types and ages of patients being seen and conditions likely encountered permits advance reading in developmental or diagnostic principles so that the student can demonstrate knowledge and be slightly more comfortable in a potentially scary setting.

YOUR TIME WITH THE STUDENT

Upon beginning a clinical experience, students need to be oriented about expectations (the teacher's and the clerkship director's), objectives, logistics (eg, where to store personal items, how to access the internet), and organization of the rotation (eg, whether students will see patients initially on their own, how much time should be taken per patient).[10] Students should be introduced to all members of the health care team; staff and nurses need to be introduced to students and oriented to their roles so that students' purpose on the team is clear.[14]

Teachers who role-model respect and concern for students' well-being and learning set the stage for success.[12] Creating a safe environment in which students can take risks (such as expanding the differential diagnoses), stretch their limits, learn, and grow is important.[4] A safe learning environment allows learners to acknowledge their attitudes and beliefs, knowledge gaps, uncertainty, and mistakes. Humility can be a powerful tool and requires open-mindedness, a willingness to consider other views, and a readiness to learn from other perspectives. Some teachers may be reluctant to say

"I don't know" or "let's look it up" for fear of appearing incompetent. A teacher's willingness to admit ignorance is a powerful way to model openness to lifelong learning and build a safe learning environment for everyone.[12]

Teachers can build a positive learning environment by avoiding interrupting students before they finish presenting a case and using good eye contact, a supportive tone of voice, and appreciative facial expressions to create students' sense of safety.[15] Humor, when used occasionally, can motivate attention and, more importantly, can foster a safe learning environment by diffusing anxiety and tension.[16]

During interactions with students, several important concepts contribute to a positive learning environment: direct observation,[17] formative feedback,[18] and open communication.[14] In addition, students generally want to progress during each clinical placement, and they appreciate when teachers create an environment that facilitates progress by providing targeted feedback, opportunities to practice the skills about which they received feedback, and then opportunities to demonstrate progress to their teachers.[19] While together with the student (whether during an emergency department shift, a few days on the wards, or several months in clinic) teachers can enhance the learning environment by being positive role models[12] and treating students as meaningful members of the health care team.[14]

AT THE COMPLETION OF YOUR TIME WITH STUDENTS

Upon completion of a shift or rotation, great clinical teachers reflect with their students to review learning points and logistical issues.[20] Importantly, great clinical teachers provide relevant and meaningful summative feedback and offer concrete suggestions on how students may improve.[18] The great clinical teacher also asks for feedback, for example, by asking, "how could I have made this experience more effective for you?" Discussing how concepts learned by students will enhance their future medical practice will complete the learning cycle in a positive environment.

CONCLUSIONS

Great clinical teachers take deliberate actions to foster a positive learning environment. They recognize that making the clinical setting feel safe, welcoming, and open will lead to greater learning and enhanced patient care. They appreciate that the students will, in the not-too-distant future, be their colleagues, and they treat them with the respect and support they deserve. Ultimately, the learning environment enriches the effect of the teacher.

REFERENCES

1. Bannister SL, Raszka WV Jr, Maloney CG. What makes a great clinical teacher in pediatrics? Lessons learned from the literature. *Pediatrics*. 2010;125(5). Available at: www.pediatrics.org/cgi/content/full/125/5/e863

2. Dudas RA, Bannister SL. It's not just what you know: the non-cognitive attributes of great clinical teachers. *Pediatrics*. 2014;134(5). Available at: www.pediatrics.org/cgi/content/full/134/5/e852

3. Genn JM. AMEE Medical Education Guide No. 23 (Part 1): Curriculum, environment, climate, quality and change in medical education: a unifying perspective. *Med Teach*. 2001a;23(4):337–344

4. Huang SL. Learning environments at higher education institutions: relationships with academic aspirations and satisfaction. *Learn Environ Res*. 2012;15(3):363–378 10.1007/s10984-012-9114-6

5. Wayne SJ, Fortner SA, Kitzes JA, Timm C, Kalishman S. Cause or effect? The relationship between student perception of the medical school learning environment and academic performance on USMLE Step 1. *Med Teach*. 2013;35(5):376–380

6. Branch WT Jr. Supporting the moral development of medical students. *J Gen Intern Med*. 2000;15(7):503–508 10.1046/j.1525-1497.2000.06298.x

7. Shochet RB, Colbert-Getz JM, Levine RB, Wright SM. Gauging events that influence students' perceptions of the medical school learning environment: findings from one institution. *Acad Med*. 2013;88(2):246–252

8. AAMC Statement on the Learning Environment. Washington, DC: AAMC; 2014. Available at: https://www.aamc.org/initiatives/learningenvironment/. Accessed April 3, 2015

9. Feudtner C, Christakis DA, Christakis NA. Do clinical clerks suffer ethical erosion? Students' perceptions of their ethical environment and personal development. *Acad Med*. 1994;69(8):670–679

10. Raszka WV Jr, Maloney CG, Hanson JL. Getting off to a good start: discussing goals and expectations with medical students. *Pediatrics*. 2010;126(2). Available at: www.pediatrics.org/cgi/content/full/126/2/e193

11. Graffam B. Active learning in medical education: strategies for beginning implementation. *Med Teach*. 2007;29(1):38–42

12. Passi V, Johnson S, Peile E, Wright S, Hafferty F, Johnson N. Doctor role modelling in medical education: BEME Guide No. 27. *Med Teach*. 2013;35(9):e1422–e1436

13. Miller S, LoFromento MA, Curtis J. (2006) COMSEP Pediatric Physical Examination [Video file]. Available at: mms://129.106.144.1/archive/ms/pedi/PDPhysical.wmv

14. Bannister SL, Wickenheiser HM, Keegan DA. Key elements of highly effective teams. *Pediatrics*. 2014;133(2). Available at: www.pediatrics.org/cgi/content/full/133/2/e184

15. Karani R, Fromme HB, Cayea D, Muller D, Schwartz A, Harris IB. How medical students learn from residents in the workplace: a qualitative study. *Acad Med*. 2014;89(3):490–496

16. Poirier TI, Wilhelm M. Use of humor to enhance learning: bull's eye or off the mark. *Am J Pharm Educ*. 2014;78(2):27

17. Hanson JL, Bannister SL, Clark A, Raszka WV Jr. Oh, what can you see: the role of observation in medical student education. *Pediatrics* 2010;126(5).

Available at: www.pediatrics.org/cgi/content/full/126/5/e843

18. Gigante J, Dell M, Sharkey A. Getting beyond "good job": how to give effective feedback. *Pediatrics*. 2011;127(2). Available at: www.pediatrics.org/cgi/content/full/127/2/e205

19. Seltz LB, Montgomery A, Lane JL, Soep J, Hanson JL. Medical students' experiences working with frequently rotating pediatric inpatient attending physicians. *Hosp Pediatr*. 2014;4(4): 239–246

20. Murdoch-Eaton D, Sandars J. Reflection: moving from a mandatory ritual to meaningful professional development. *Arch Dis Child*. 2014;99(3):279–283

21. Roff S, McAleer S, Harden RM, et al. Development and validation of the Dundee Ready Education Environment Measure (DREEM). *Med Teach*. 1997; 19(4):295–299

22. Dornan T, Muijtjens A, Graham J, Scherpbier A, Boshuizen H. Manchester Clinical Placement Index (MCPI). Conditions for medical students' learning in hospital and community placements. *Adv Health Sci Educ Theory Pract*. 2012;17(5):703–716

23. Schönrock-Adema J, Bouwkamp-Timmer T, van Hell EA, Cohen-Schotanus J. Key elements in assessing the educational environment: where is the theory? *Adv Health Sci Educ Theory Pract*. 2012;17(5):727–742

24. Long M, Blankenburg R, Butani L. Questioning as a teaching tool. *Pediatrics*. 2015;135(3):406–408. Available at: www.pediatrics.org/cgi/content/full/135/3/e406

A Little Hurts a Lot: Exploring the Impact of Microaggressions in Pediatric Medical Education

Kimberly Young, MSc,ᵃ Angela Punnett, MD, FRCPC,ᵇ,ᶜ Shazeen Suleman, MSc, MD, MPH, FRCPCᶜ,ᵈ,ᵉ

"You have such a difficult name."

"You speak English so well!"

"Do you really eat bats?"

When Faiza, an adolescent patient, is told by her doctor that her name is difficult to pronounce, she hears, "You are different, and you don't belong." When a patient tells Christopher, a resident, that he speaks English really well, he wonders what assumptions they have made regarding his ability to be a good physician. When Kimberly, a medical student of Chinese heritage, is asked by her patient if she eats "strange foods" during the current coronavirus disease 2019 pandemic, she feels the sting of heightened xenophobia. Although possibly seeming benign, these incidents are the definition of microaggressions, like "death by a thousand cuts."

WHAT ARE MICROAGGRESSIONS?

Microaggressions, as suggested by the prefix, are not overt or grandiose displays of discrimination.[1] They are inherently nuanced discriminatory remarks or behaviors stemming from unconscious bias, often unintentional on the part of the aggressor. Although we focus on racist microaggressions in this article, many groups may experience them, including differently abled individuals, sexual and gender minorities, and religious minorities.[2] The subtle nature of microaggressions makes them difficult to identify and address for involved parties. Yet their damage is real and widespread, impacting medical trainees' learning, work performance, and even career decisions.[3] Thus, the learning environment may mirror harassment and discrimination that exist in society.

MICROAGGRESSIONS IN THE LEARNING ENVIRONMENT

The learning environment in pediatric medical education involves a number of participants: a learner (ie, a medical student or resident), an educator (ie, an attending physician, a resident, or an allied health care professional), and a caregiver, yet it is always patient centered. These relationships mean that the impact of the microaggression extends beyond the direct recipient: there is an impressionable child, youth, or student internalizing these exchanges as examples of the world around them. Microaggressions are not bounded by status and can be bidirectional; they can be inflicted by educators on learners, caregivers on learners, educators on caregivers, or educators on educators. The way these interactions are ignored or addressed sends a silent, but powerful, message to the child,

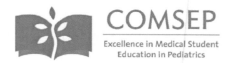

COMSEP
Excellence in Medical Student
Education in Pediatrics

ᶜDepartment of Pediatrics and ᵃFaculty of Medicine, University of Toronto, Toronto, Ontario, Canada; ᵇDepartment of Pediatrics, The Hospital for Sick Children, Toronto, Ontario, Canada; ᵈWomen and Children's Health, Unity Health Toronto and St. Michael's Hospital, Toronto, Ontario, Canada; and ᵉLi Ka Shing Knowledge Institute, St. Michael's Hospital, Toronto, Ontario, Canada

As coauthors, we bring a diverse range of perspectives rooted in our identities and lived experiences. Ms Young (she and her) is a Chinese-Canadian senior medical student leader at the University of Toronto; Dr Punnett (she and her) is a white-Canadian pediatric oncologist and Director of Undergraduate Medical Education (Pediatrics) at the University of Toronto; Dr Suleman (she and her) is an Indo-Canadian Muslim pediatrician and Assistant Professor at the University of Toronto (Pediatrics); and all authors contributed equally to the conceptualization, drafting, and revision of the manuscript, approved the final manuscript as submitted, and agree to be accountable for all aspects of the work.

DOI: https://doi.org/10.1542/peds.2020-1636

Accepted for publication Apr 24, 2020

Address correspondence to Shazeen Suleman, MSc, MD, MPH, FRCPC, Women and Children's Health, Unity Health Toronto, St. Michael's Hospital, 30 Bond St, 15 Cardinal Carter - Room 014, Toronto, ON, Canada M5B 1W8. E-mail: shazeen.suleman@unityhealth.to

PEDIATRICS (ISSN Numbers: Print, 0031-4005; Online, 1098-4275).

FINANCIAL DISCLOSURE: The authors have indicated they have no financial relationships relevant to this article to disclose.

FUNDING: No external funding.

POTENTIAL CONFLICT OF INTEREST: The authors have indicated they have no potential conflicts of interest to disclose.

To cite: Young K, Punnett A, Suleman S. A Little Hurts a Lot: Exploring the Impact of Microaggressions in Pediatric Medical Education. *Pediatrics.* 2020;146(1):e20201636

youth, or student about what is acceptable and whether they are accepted in the world. The impact of discrimination on child health is significant, from worsening mental health to high-risk behaviors[4,5] and it is paramount that as pediatric educators, our learning environment does not contribute to this.

Unfortunately, microaggressions in medical education remain a daily reality for many trainees. At vulnerable stages in their careers, these negative encounters may leave trainees with a sense of "otherness," reinforcing a feeling that they do not fit the archetype of a certain specialty, setting, or medicine broadly. Moreover, trainees are tasked with building resiliency and maintaining wellness in a milieu that not only fails to evolve with them but provides repeated insults to their self-worth. Similarly, although society places physicians in positions of privilege, physicians from marginalized groups regularly experience microaggressions, themselves. Microaggressions may erode a sense of self-efficacy,[6] blunting the trajectory of rising clinician leaders and educators, further perpetuating the homogeneity among medical faculty. For both learners and health care professionals alike, the damage inflicted by microaggressions is pervasive and potent, associated with increased depression, anxiety, and trauma.[6-8] We must make a commitment to support one another; a more-unified and tolerant medical community not only promotes wellness among health care professionals but may also improve health outcomes for patients.[9]

Microaggressions have become so ubiquitous that it can be difficult for those affected to speak out about each isolated event without seeming overly sensitive. Although resilience helps trainees navigate some of the challenges they will face in medicine, we cannot call on students to mitigate these encounters with coping strategies alone. Clinical educators can serve as powerful allies to support and empower trainees who are experiencing mistreatment. Yet, although many teachers feel compelled to answer this call to action, they may also feel ill-equipped to translate those feelings into practice. It is critical to train all educators and learners to prepare for, recognize, and respond to microaggressions to mitigate their effect and provide a supportive learning and practice environment for our teams and patients (Fig 1).

OPPORTUNITIES FOR EDUCATORS

First, we recommend that all learners and educators receive formal education about explicit and structural racism and discrimination and be encouraged to engage in candid personal and group reflections on their historical underpinnings and modern manifestations. Many institutions now recommend training to identify one's own implicit associations or bias.[10] Group reflections allow for the sharing of lived experiences of microaggressions and can help staff and learners practice potential responses.

Second, we urge clinical educators to take responsibility within the clinical context to identify and address microaggressions in the moment, naming the behavior as inappropriate and refocusing the interaction to the professional context for the actor and any involved trainees. These in-the-moment interventions can be done respectfully by directly reframing a response. In Kimberly's case above, if witnessed by the educator, they can refocus the interaction on the patient's immediate needs; this pivot may also draw the patient's attention to the inappropriate nature of their remark. After this, the educator should debrief the interaction with the trainee in a neutral, safe space to provide support and acknowledge the impact of the microaggression.

EDUCATOR-LEARNER OPPORTUNITIES

Beyond addressing witnessed interactions, we believe educators should create spaces for trainees and educators alike to disclose experiences of microaggressions, whether this occurred as the recipient or the actor. Critical reflection around the impact of the interaction encourages analyses of behaviors,[11] helping to shift the onus away from expecting trainees to suppress reactions when facing discrimination and, instead, placing responsibility

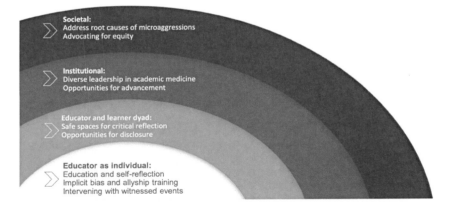

FIGURE 1

An approach to addressing microaggressions in medical education. Strategies at the individual, educator-learner dyad, institutional, and societal levels may support the mitigation of micro-aggressions in medical education.

on educators to increase their sensitivity and awareness. After all, each of us can control what we ourselves say, but others cannot control what they hear or how it makes them feel.

OPPORTUNITIES FOR INSTITUTIONS AND SOCIETY

Third, we strongly recommend increasing diversity within medical education leadership, such that more individuals in positions of power share the experiences of their trainees. It is important to build relationships to create solidarity with marginalized groups, in other words, to become an ally. However, it is impossible to respond to a transgression when you are unable to recognize it. Because microaggressions are subtle, the progress we stand to make through our allies is often limited by their lack of lived experiences. Currently, the demographics of academic pediatric leadership does not reflect their learners or the general population.[12,13] One way to increase diversity is by explicitly valuing different strengths and experiences in academic medicine, particularly in candidates being considered for recruitment and advancement. Increasing pressure on medical faculty to excel solely in research effectively minimizes the importance of excellence in teaching, clinical service, and advocacy.[14] With an ever-evolving scope of practice, we believe that our institutions must consider the broad definition of academic scholarship to give merit to less-tangible, although equally significant, means of productivity; for example, community leadership and engagement.[15] Finally, both educators and learners can strive to address the root causes of microaggressions and advocate for a more-equitable society.

CONCLUSIONS

In an increasingly pluralistic world, we can look to a future when microaggressions are acknowledged, addressed, and ultimately no longer exist. In our previous examples, Faiza would be asked how best to pronounce her name, Christopher would be praised for his bedside clinical skills, and Kimberly would feel empowered after her preceptor's intervention. It is this world that we want our patients to see and our learners to grow in and one that we can achieve with a concerted effort to acknowledge, identify, and address.

REFERENCES

1. Wong G, Derthick AO, David EJR, Saw A, Okazaki S. The what, the why, and the how: a review of racial microaggressions research in psychology. *Race Soc Probl*. 2014;6(2):181–200

2. Sue DW. Microaggressions: more than just race. *Psychology Today*. November 17, 2010. Available at: https://www.psychologytoday.com/ca/blog/microaggressions-in-everyday-life/201011/microaggressions-more-just-race. Accessed March 11, 2020

3. Stratton TD, McLaughlin MA, Witte FM, Fosson SE, Nora LM. Does students' exposure to gender discrimination and sexual harassment in medical school affect specialty choice and residency program selection? *Acad Med*. 2005;80(4):400–408

4. Shepherd CCJ, Li J, Cooper MN, Hopkins KD, Farrant BM. The impact of racial discrimination on the health of Australian Indigenous children aged 5-10 years: analysis of national longitudinal data. *Int J Equity Health*. 2017;16(1):116

5. Sittner Hartshorn KJ, Whitbeck LB, Hoyt DR. Exploring the relationships of perceived discrimination, anger, and aggression among North American Indigenous adolescents. *Soc Ment Health*. 2012;2(1):53–67

6. Wong-Padoongpatt G, Zane N, Okazaki S, Saw A. Decreases in implicit self-esteem explain the racial impact of microaggressions among Asian Americans. *J Couns Psychol*. 2017;64(5):574–583

7. Torres L, Driscoll MW, Burrow AL. Racial microaggressions and psychological functioning among highly achieving African-Americans: a mixed-methods approach. *J Soc Clin Psychol*. 2010;29:1074–1099

8. Huynh VW. Ethnic microaggressions and the depressive and somatic symptoms of Latino and Asian American adolescents. *J Youth Adolesc*. 2012;41(7):831–846

9. Suleman S, Garber KD, Rutkow L. Xenophobia as a determinant of health: an integrative review. *J Public Health Policy*. 2018;39(4):407–423

10. Harvard University. Project Implicit preliminary information. 2011. Available at: https://implicit.harvard.edu/implicit/takeatest.html. Accessed March 27, 2020

11. Overland MK, Zumsteg JM, Lindo EG, et al. Microaggressions in clinical training and practice. *PM R*. 2019;11(9):1004–1012

12. Mendoza FS, Walker LR, Stoll BJ, et al. Diversity and inclusion training in pediatric departments. *Pediatrics*. 2015;135(4):707–713

13. Kaplan SH, Sullivan LM, Dukes KA, Phillips CF, Kelch RP, Schaller JG. Sex differences in academic advancement. Results of a national study of pediatricians. *N Engl J Med*. 1996;335(17):1282–1289

14. Schimanski LA, Alperin JP. The evaluation of scholarship in academic promotion and tenure processes: past, present, and future. *F1000 Res*. 2018;7:1605

15. Boyer EL. From scholarship reconsidered to scholarship assessed. *Quest*. 1996;48(2):129–139

Taking Humanism Back to the Bedside

Jennifer Plant, MD, MEd[a], Michael A. Barone, MD, MPH[b], Janet R. Serwint, MD[b], Lavjay Butani, MD, MACM[a]

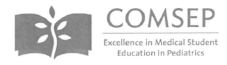

Excellence in Medical Student
Education in Pediatrics

[a]Department of Pediatrics, University of California, Davis,
Sacramento, California; and [b]Department of Pediatrics,
Johns Hopkins University School of Medicine, Baltimore,
Maryland

Drs Plant, Barone, and Serwint drafted part of the
initial manuscript and edited the entire manuscript;
Dr Butani conceptualized the manuscript, drafted
part of the initial manuscript, and edited the entire
manuscript; and all authors approved the final
manuscript as submitted.

www.pediatrics.org/cgi/doi/10.1542/peds.2015-3042

DOI: 10.1542/peds.2015-3042

Accepted for publication Aug 17, 2015

Address correspondence to Jennifer Plant, MD, MEd,
Department of Pediatrics, University of California,
Davis, 2516 Stockton Blvd, Sacramento, CA 95817.
E-mail: jplant@ucdavis.edu

PEDIATRICS (ISSN Numbers: Print, 0031-4005; Online,
1098-4275).

FINANCIAL DISCLOSURE: The authors have indicated
they have no financial relationships relevant to this
article to disclose.

FUNDING: No external funding.

POTENTIAL CONFLICT OF INTEREST: The authors have
indicated they have no potential conflicts of interest
to disclose.

After attending The Arnold P. Gold Foundation's "Barriers to Sustaining Humanism in Medicine" symposium in 1996, Steve Miller and Richard Sarkin proposed a Traveling Fellows program for the foundation. The program was approved, and Steve and Rich served as the program's 2 Traveling Fellows until their untimely death on October 19, 2004. Steve and Rich, both Council on Medical Student Education in Pediatrics presidents known for their creativity and charisma, brought to our collective consciousness the need to promote humanism in our work as clinicians, teachers, and role models. When they died, Steve's Chair at Columbia, John Driscoll, urged that their memory be honored by devoting time each October to promoting humanism.[1] It is in this spirit that COMSEP Perspectives provides the following article.
– Kenneth B. Roberts, MD

WHAT IS HUMANISM?

Reflecting on our journey through medicine, we may recall pivotal moments that re-affirmed our commitment to the values of our profession. These moments may relate to the spirit of discovery inherent in the practice of medicine, to the recognition afforded by society to medical practitioners, or to service toward those who are suffering and in need of care. This last attribute, which encompasses a spirit of sincere concern for the centrality of human values in every aspect of professional activity, is referred to as humanism.[2] Humanism is a way of being defined by the characteristics of empathy, altruism, and compassion.[3] As so eloquently stated by Sir William Osler, "it is much more important to know what sort of person has a disease, than to know what sort of disease a person has."[4]

WHY PRACTICE AND TEACH HUMANISM?

The literature demonstrates that patients cared for by humanistic clinicians have better outcomes,[5] increased satisfaction,[6] and improved adherence to an agreed-upon plan of care.[7] When coupled with the observations highlighting the decline of empathy among learners[8] and the missed opportunities for demonstrating empathy among practicing physicians,[9] it becomes essential for us to consciously role model and teach humanistic values to learners. Fortunately, the medical literature provides supporting evidence that the construct of humanism can be learned and taught.[10]

ATTRIBUTES OF HUMANISTIC TEACHERS

Today's health care environment poses challenges to a practice founded on humanism. Exponential advances in medical technology, documentation demands, and an increasing emphasis on the clinical productivity and the business aspects of medicine have the potential to distance physicians from their patients.[11] Recognizing the potential impact of these challenges, we, as educators, need to maintain the focus on humanistic practices. In 2014, Chou et al[12] examined the attitudes and behaviors of highly humanistic physicians. Her team found that attitudes of humanism include humility (cherishing the privilege and responsibility that society has bestowed upon us), curiosity (a genuine desire to know about the people we interact with), and a desire to maintain high standards of behavior.

Behaviors that have helped educators maintain these attitudes include self-reflection, seeking connections with patients, a focus on personal resilience and wellness, and teaching and role modeling humanistic care. Intentionally practicing these behaviors and creating an environment with a focus on humanism can hold teachers accountable, help maintain humanism, and ensure that we role model humanism for our learners.

A FRAMEWORK FOR TEACHING HUMANISM

Steven Miller and Hillary Schmidt proposed that the practice and teaching of humanism could be conceptualized by using a framework, similar to the approach for the physical examination or creation of a differential diagnosis. Their article, "The Habit of Humanism: A Framework for Making Humanistic Care a Reflexive Clinical Skill," posits that humanism can become a habit by practicing 3 steps: (1) identifying perspectives of the patient, the patient's loved ones, and the health care provider; (2) reflecting on how these perspectives converge or conflict; and (3) choosing to act altruistically by endorsing and understanding the perspectives of the patient and family.[13]

There are numerous teaching strategies that build on this framework to promote humanism in daily medical practice.[14] Many strategies are embedded during the practice of providing care to patients while others can be taught outside of a patient-care setting, as outlined in Table 1.[15–19]

SUMMARY

A quotation by George Eliot in *Middlemarch* summarizes everyday humanism:

We do not expect people to be deeply moved by what is not unusual. That

TABLE 1 Teaching Strategies

Clinical Practice Recommendation	Examples
Strategies embedded during patient care activities	
Encourage learners to incorporate humanism into personal learning goals and individualized learning plans	"I want to explore and address the fears expressed by the parents/guardians of the patients I see"
Promote perspective taking, the act of viewing a situation from others' points of view, by asking learners to explore the perspectives of the patient, the family, and the health care team	"What do you think is the patient's most important current priority? Why? What is your point of view on that? What do you see as your priority and role?"
Heighten learner awareness regarding the potential impact of illness	"Did it surprise you when that patient's mother became upset when you told her that her child has a lung infection? Why do you think she became so emotional?"
Incorporate psychosocial aspects of patients' stories into presentations	Encourage learners to spend 5 min getting to know their patients and families as people, rather than as patients, and share this information with the team
Refer to patients and parents by their actual names, not as their diagnoses[15] and not necessarily as "Mom" or "Dad"	Role model for learners how to ask family members how they would like to be addressed by the health care team
Practice family/patient-centered rounds that include active participation of the patient and family in the discussion and decision-making process	Include introductions, meeting and acknowledging all members of the family and team
	Ensure that presentations are directed toward the patient/family and do not use medical jargon
	Consider having the main presenter seated next to the patient and family member
	Explicitly give family members permission to interrupt rounds when they have any modifications to the history, questions, concerns, or things to add
"Reflect on action" on impactful events as they occur	Share emotional impact of patients' stories on your own self
	Acknowledge your individual struggles
	Use opportunities to teach when encounters could have been more humanistic[16]
"Reflect on action" after impactful events have occurred: capture the opportunity to reflect on seminal events by debriefing after patient encounters that have a powerful impact[17]	Use a debriefing framework such as Welcome and introductions Factual information and case review Grief responses and other emotions Strategies for coping with grief Lessons learned Conclusion[18]
Facilitate end of day/week/rotation reflection	"What did you learn about your patients today?" "Here are the names of our patients that we cared for this week. What did they teach you? What will you remember? What do you recall about these patients as people?"
Structured activities independent of direct patient care	
Engage in experiences with graphic, fine, and performance arts to facilitate "enstrangement" (making the familiar unfamiliar) and viewing what may have become mundane with a keener vision[19]	Visit a museum; discuss a piece of art, poem, or video
	Ask learners to take on the roles of the subjects or characters and share their feelings and emotional reactions to the events described
	Debrief on how perspectives may differ from person to person yet all are valuable
Use trigger videos or movie clips	Watch and discuss *Use of Empathy: The Human Connection to Patient Care* created by the Cleveland Clinic (https://www.youtube.com/watch?v=cDDWvj_q-o8)

TABLE 1 Continued

Clinical Practice Recommendation	Examples
Use narratives to stimulate discussion	Distribute selected works from such series as The Journal of the American Medical Association's *A Piece of My Mind*
Gain better understanding of patients in the context of their family, cultural and spiritual values, and their community	Arrange a home visit of a patient or neighborhood Send learners on a tour of the neighborhood around the clinic or practice, then talk about what they saw and the implications for patient care decisions

element of tragedy which lies in the very fact of frequency has not yet wrought itself into the coarse emotion of mankind and perhaps our frames could hardly bear much of it. If we had a keen vision and feeling of all ordinary human life, it would be like hearing the grass grow and the squirrels' heartbeat, and we should die of that roar which lies on the other side of silence. As it is the quickest of us walk about well wadded with stupidity.[20]

As Eliot so eloquently states, being empathic can be considered a double-edged sword; while it facilitates the opening of oneself to others' perspectives and emotions with the purpose of understanding them and caring for them better, it can also lead to our bearing a heavy burden. There should remain little doubt, however, that empathic actions are a core part of the virtue of humanism and must be practiced and taught, both implicitly and explicitly. Our hope is that by using Miller and Schmidt's framework on the "habit" of humanism[13] and the various educational strategies outlined here, a great clinical teacher can channel his or her innermost humanistic attributes as a role model and overcome perceived barriers. Such actions could only further improve the care we provide and foster humanism in our learners.

ACKNOWLEDGMENT

The authors thank Dr Kenneth B. Roberts for his poignant remembrances of Drs Miller and Sarkin as well as his inspiration to promote humanism in medical education.

REFERENCES

1. Driscoll JM. Steven Miller, MD, and Richard Sarkin, MD: men for other. *J Pediatr.* 2006;148(1):1–2

2. Pelligrino ED. *Humanism and the Physician.* Knoxville, TN: The University of Tennessee Press; 1979

3. Cohen JJ. Viewpoint: linking professionalism to humanism: what it means, why it matters. *Acad Med.* 2007; 82(11):1029–1032

4. Silverman ME, Murray TJ, Bryan CS. *The Quotable Osler.* Philadelphia, PA: American College of Physicians; 2007

5. Hojat M, Louis DZ, Markham FW, Wender R, Rabinowitz C, Gonnella JS. Physicians' empathy and clinical outcomes for diabetic patients. *Acad Med.* 2011;86(3): 359–364

6. Steinhausen S, Ommen O, Antoine SL, Koehler T, Pfaff H, Neugebauer E. Short- and long-term subjective medical treatment outcome of trauma surgery patients: the importance of physician empathy. *Patient Prefer Adherence.* 2014;8:1239–1253

7. Sylvia LG, Hay A, Ostacher MJ, et al. Association between therapeutic alliance, care satisfaction, and pharmacological adherence in bipolar disorder. *J Clin Psychopharmacol.* 2013; 33(3):343–350

8. Hojat M, Vergare MJ, Maxwell K, et al. The devil is in the third year: a longitudinal study of erosion of empathy in medical school. *Acad Med.* 2009;84(9):1182–1191

9. Morse DS, Edwardsen EA, Gordon HS. Missed opportunities for interval empathy in lung cancer communication. *Arch Intern Med.* 2008;168(17):1853–1858

10. Misra-Hebert AD, Isaacson JH, Kohn M, et al. Improving empathy of physicians through guided reflective writing. *Int J Med Educ.* 2012;3:71–77

11. Cruess RL, Cruess SR, Steinert Y, eds. *Teaching Medical Professionalism.* New York: Cambridge University Press; 2009

12. Chou CM, Kellom K, Shea JA. Attitudes and habits of highly humanistic physicians. *Acad Med.* 2014;89(9):1252–1258

13. Miller SZ, Schmidt HJ. The habit of humanism: a framework for making humanistic care a reflexive clinical skill. *Acad Med.* 1999;74(7):800–803

14. Branch WT Jr, Kern D, Haidet P, et al. The patient-physician relationship. Teaching the human dimensions of care in clinical settings. *JAMA.* 2001;286(9): 1067–1074

15. Roberts KB. Children and their diseases. *Arch Pediatr Adolesc Med.* 1995;149(5):583

16. Novack DH, Epstein RM, Paulsen RH. Toward creating physician-healers: fostering medical students' self-awareness, personal growth, and well-being. *Acad Med.* 1999;74(5):516–520

17. Treadway K. The code. *N Engl J Med.* 2007;357(13):1273–1275

18. Keene EA, Hutton N, Hall B, Rushton C. Bereavement debriefing sessions: an intervention to support health care professionals in managing their grief after the death of a patient. *Pediatr Nurs.* 2010;36(4):185–189, quiz 190

19. Kumagai AK, Wear D. "Making strange": a role for the humanities in medical education. *Acad Med.* 2014;89(7):973–977

20. Eliot G. *Middlemarch.* Hertfordshire, England: Wordsworth Editions; 1994

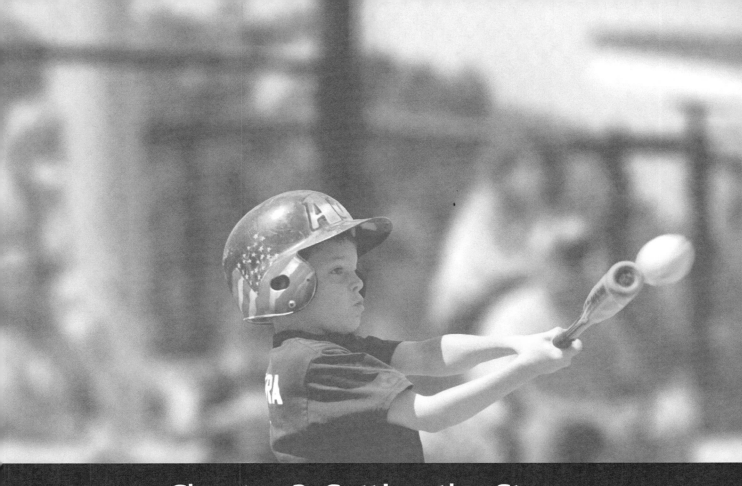

Chapter 2: Setting the Stage

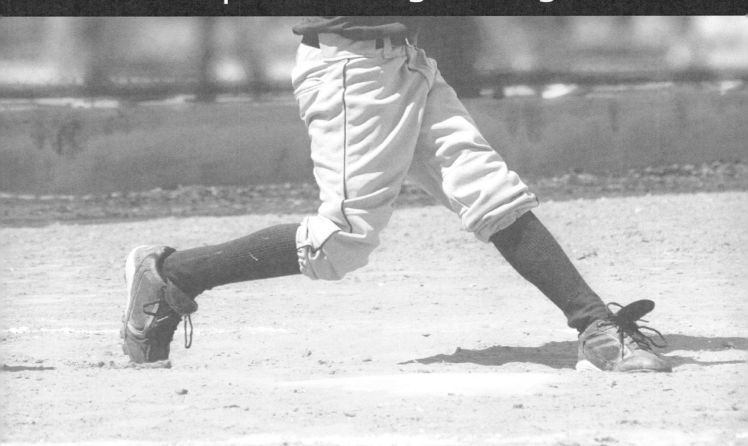

Chapter 2

Setting the Stage for Great Clinical Learning

By Sandra M Sanguino, MD, MPH
Associate Professor of Pediatrics and Medical Education, Northwestern University Feinberg School of Medicine

Learning in the clinical environment is challenging. Students are expected to help provide medical care to patients while simultaneously mastering an ever-expanding body of knowledge. If we are to ensure the success of our learners, we need to make sure they are adequately prepared to enter this complicated learning environment. One way to help prepare our learners is to "set the stage." What does this mean? Setting the stage is "to create conditions in which something is likely to happen."[1] The "something" we want to happen is learning.

Early in training, students are taught how to conduct patient-centered interviews. The first step learners are taught is how set the stage.[2] Students are taught various techniques that allow for the establishment of the patient-clinician relationship and ensure a patient-centered atmosphere. Similarly, if we want to establish a learner-centered atmosphere to enable our students to thrive, we need to be deliberate about how we set the stage for learning in the complicated clinical environment.

The 5 articles in this chapter discuss how we can help set the stage for our learners.

In the first article, "Getting Off to a Good Start: Discussing Goals and Expectations with Medical Students," we are reminded that the first day of clinical rotations can be particularly challenging for medical students for a variety of reasons.[3] Raszka et al provide a framework for orienting students to the clinical setting. Providing students with a thorough orientation can help set the stage for a supportive and effective learning environment.

Understanding how to effectively work as a team is critically important to the delivery of health care. Effective teams decrease length of stay, improve coordination of care, increase patient satisfaction, and improve health outcomes.[4] The authors of the next article featured in this chapter identified 3 key elements for effective teams: purpose, openness, and roles and skills.[5] By clearly outlining the expectations of the team, learners have a road map to help navigate the complexities of working in a team environment.

Our learners often work in clinical environments where there are many levels of trainees: medical students, residents, fellows. The article by Quigley et al outlines a novel way to engage multilevel learner groups in the clinical setting.[6] The ENGAGE mnemonic (Everyone teaches, Novel topics, Guide, Ascend the ladder, Groups within the group, Empower learners for autonomy) provides preceptors with tools to engage learners at all levels. By utilizing these strategies, skilled clinical teachers can meet the needs of the individual learners.

In the next piece in this series, a model for coaching called Clinical COACH (Contract, Optimize, Act, Check-In) is presented.[7] In Step 1 of this model, the learner and the coach develop an understanding of the coaching relationship. This allows the learner to identify goals and helps set the stage for the success of the student in the learning environment.

The final paper in this section provides an overview of Entrustable Professional Activities (EPAs).[8] The authors describe how EPAs provide a framework for describing the work that physicians do and the skills that medical students must acquire before graduation from medical school. The EPA framework provides students with an understanding of what is expected, which will allow students to set goals for their learning.

This collection of articles provides teachers with various ways to help set the stage for learning. By deliberately employing strategies to set the stage, outstanding clinical teachers can help optimize the learning environment and set students up for success.

References

1. https://www.macmillandictionary.com/us/dictionary/american/set-the-stage-for-something
2. Chapter 3. the beginning of the interview: patient-centered interviewing. Fortin A.H., VI, & Dwamena F.C., & Frankel R.M., & Smith R.C.(Eds.), (2012). *Smith's Patient-Centered Interviewing: An Evidence-Based Method, 3e*. McGraw-Hill. https://accessmedicine.mhmedical.com/content.aspx?bookid=501&sectionid=41021119
3. Raszka WV, Maloney CG, Hanson JL. Getting off to a good start: Discussing goals & expectations with medical students. *Pediatrics* 2010;126:193-195.
4. Mickan SM. Evaluating the effectiveness of health care teams. *Aust Health Rev.* 2005:29(2) 211-217.
5. Bannister SL, Wickenheiser HM, Keegan DA. Key elements of highly effective teams. *Pediatrics.* 2014 Feb;133(2):184-6. doi: 10.1542/peds.2013-3734.
6. Quigley PD, Potisek NM, Barone MA. How to "ENGAGE" Multilevel Learner Groups in the Clinical Setting. *Pediatrics.* 2017 Nov;140(5):e20172861. doi: 10.1542/peds.2017-2861.
7. Bannister SL, Wu TF, Keegan DA. The Clinical COACH: How to Enable Your Learners to Own Their Learning. *Pediatrics.* 2018 Nov;142(5):e20182601. doi: 10.1542/peds.2018-2601.
8. Hanson JL, Bannister SL. To Trust or Not to Trust? An Introduction to Entrustable Professional Activities. *Pediatrics.* 2016 Nov;138(5):e20162373. doi: 10.1542/peds.2016-2373.

PEDIATRICS PERSPECTIVES

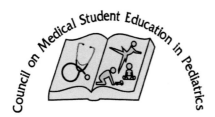

CONTRIBUTORS: William V. Raszka Jr, MD,[a] Christopher G. Maloney, MD, PhD,[b] and Janice L. Hanson, PhD, EdS[c]
[a]Department of Pediatrics, University of Vermont College of Medicine, Burlington, Vermont; [b]Department of Pediatrics, University of Utah, Salt Lake City, Utah; and [c]Departments of Medicine and Pediatrics, Uniformed Services University of the Health Sciences, Bethesda, Maryland

Address correspondence to William V. Raszka Jr, MD, Department of Pediatrics, University of Vermont College of Medicine, Given Courtyard, Burlington, VT 05405. E-mail: william.raszka@uvm.edu

Accepted for publication May 20, 2010

doi:10.1542/peds.2010-1439

Getting Off to a Good Start: Discussing Goals and Expectations With Medical Students

The next several articles by the Council on Medical Student Education in Pediatrics (COMSEP) will describe the strategies and skills that great clinical teachers use to enhance medical student learning, regardless of the clinical setting, and illustrate ways to incorporate these strategies and skills into daily practice. This article begins the series and explores the role of orientation to a learning environment.

We all remember the first day of a clinical rotation during medical school or residency or even the first day of a new job. We wanted to know important information to help prepare us for the experience. An orientation should align the expectations of the student, preceptor, and educational program to help create a successful and enjoyable learning environment. Medical students face a particularly difficult challenge, because they usually begin their clinical experiences in pediatrics with no knowledge of a particular office or clinic and limited clinical experience with children. Furthermore, the preceptor rarely knows the student and usually did not design the educational curriculum, which creates a tenuous beginning for the student-preceptor relationship. Yet, by the end of the clinical experience, the student is expected to accomplish certain tasks and the preceptor must submit an evaluation of the student. One of the most common suggestions that medical students offer preceptors is that they spend time orienting students.[1]

ORIENTATION IN CLINICAL PRACTICE During orientation, a preceptor introduces the student to the mechanics and processes of the health care team. Mechanics describe the

facilities, working hours, patient flow, and duties, among others. Processes provide the framework for learning through explicit expectations, clearly defined performance standards, and assessment. Because clinical teaching occurs in a variety of settings and for variable amounts of time, no single orientation fits all settings. For example, orientation for a student beginning a 4-week primary care block will include more information and take longer than one for a student spending a single day with a pediatric subspecialist. During orientation, the student learns about the clinical experience and the preceptor learns about the student, which equips them to tailor the educational experience to best meet the needs of the academic institution and the learner.

ORIENTATION TO THE MECHANICS OF THE TEACHING SITE Most physicians know the importance of the first encounter and, hence, rarely assign a surly employee to greet patients. The importance of the first encounter with medical students is no less important. A timely and enthusiastic welcome captures students' attention and excites them about learning.[2] Conversely, allowing a student to wait in the reception area while the staff tries to figure out what to do conveys lack of interest and preparation. For example, in a clinic, introducing the student to all members of the health care team including the receptionists, schedulers, and nurses helps them feel part of the team.[3] Beyond introductions, the student will need to know basic information about where they are to be, including what time they should arrive, where they may park (if applicable), what time they may leave, how they will be assigned patients, who they should contact if they need to be absent, whether they should attend non–clinic-based or office-based clinical activities (eg, to deliveries, school-based clinics, or conferences), how to access the Internet, and how to use the electronic medical record (if applicable). If the preceptor responsible for the student cannot orient him or her to the mechanics of the teaching site, an able assistant or colleague may do so.[4]

ORIENTATION TO THE PROCESS OF THE TEACHING SITE Orientation to the process addresses how students will learn. The first step is to make sure that both the preceptor and the student are aware of the goals and objectives or competencies of the overall educational experience (eg, the clerkship). For example, the COMSEP curriculum defines the knowledge, skill, and attitude competencies expected of clerkship students by the end of their clinical rotation.[5] Simply put, these competencies inform both students and preceptors of expected achievements.[6]

The preceptor can assess a student's experience and learning needs toward achieving expected competencies by asking questions such as (1) What is your year in medical school? (2) Which clinical rotations have you completed? (3) What types of patients have you seen? (4) What areas do you want to study or improve? and (5) How do you best learn? Armed with this knowledge, the preceptor can ensure that the teaching and learning support the curriculum and that the student has an opportunity to meet all stated competencies. For example, if students by the end of the experience are expected to correctly perform the Ortolani and Barlow maneuvers, the best way to ensure that they can is by demonstrating the correct way to perform the maneuvers and then watching the students perform the maneuvers with patients.

Although the curriculum informs the preceptor and the student of expectations, adults learn best when their own needs and interests are met. To this end, successful clinical teachers ask students what they hope to learn and then help them set personally relevant educational goals.[7] Although students still need to meet the overall competencies, learning can be tailored to meet individual goals. For example, a student may want to refine communication skills with adolescents or pursue an interest in orthopedics. Because apt clinical performance depends on awareness of one's abilities and areas that require increased knowledge and skill, a preceptor also makes an important contribution by helping the student identify tasks tailored to individual learning needs. Although learners tend to either overestimate or underestimate their overall abilities, they tend to be more successful in assessing their knowledge in relation to specific tasks.[8] Supporting the student's self-reflection, helping the student identify individual goals, and providing an opportunity to meet these personal goals furthers successful lifelong learning.[4] Moreover, listening to and acting on the student's requests conveys enormous respect for the student and is one of the most appreciated attributes of great clinical teachers.[9,10]

Students value clearly defined expectations and goals.[11,12] Expectations might include how many patients each student should see, how much time a student should spend with each patient, when the preceptor will observe the student, what information students should give to a patient when seeing a patient independently, what and how clinical information should be presented to the preceptor, and what the student should include in medical documentation. Working together, the student and preceptor should agree on specific, measurable, achievable, realistic, and time-bound (SMART) cognitive, procedural, or behavioral outcomes.[6] Giving students protected time to reflect on their experiences, how they might improve, and how they will apply what they have learned to the next patient is important for quality of care and professional development.[4] The context of the teaching experience is more important to a successful clinical experience than the number of patients seen.[11,13,14]

SUMMARY Medical students highly value a learning environment in which they feel part of the health care team, their views are valued, and they make significant contributions to the care of patients.[4] An orientation that includes an enthusiastic welcome, an opportunity to get to know from where the students have come and where they want to go, and setting mutually agreeable SMART objectives helps create a supportive and effective learning environment.[10,11,15,16]

REFERENCES

1. Lie D, Boker J, Dow E, et al. Attributes of effective community preceptors for pre-clerkship medical students. *Med Teach*. 2009;31(3):251–259

2. Irby DM. Effective clinical teaching & learning: clinical teaching and the clinical teacher. Available at: www.med.cmu.ac.th/secret/meded/ct2.htm. Accessed May 5, 2010

3. Irby DM. What clinical teachers in medicine need to know. *Acad Med*. 1994;69(5):333–342

4. Greenberg L, Ottolini M. The clerkship orientation. In: Fincher RM, ed.

Guidebook for Clerkship Directors. 3rd ed. Omaha, NE: Alliance for Clinical Education; 2005

5. Council on Medical Student Education in Pediatrics. Welcome to COMSEP. Available at: www.comsep.org. Accessed May 5, 2010

6. McKimm J, Swanwick T. Setting learning objectives. *Br J Hosp Med (Lond).* 2009;70(7):406–409

7. Menachery EP, Wright SM, Howell EE, Knight AM. Physician-teacher characteristics associated with learner-centered teaching skills. *Med Teach.* 2008;30(5):e137–e144

8. Eva KW, Regehr G. Knowing when to look it up: a new conception of self-assessment ability. *Acad Med.* 2007;82(10 suppl):S81–S84

9. Sutkin G, Wagner E, Harris I, Schiffer R. What makes a good clinical teacher in medicine? A review of the literature. *Acad Med.* 2008;83(5):452–466

10. Irby DM. Teaching and learning in ambulatory care settings: a thematic review of the literature. *Acad Med.* 1995;70(10):898–931

11. Goertzen J, Stewart M, Weston W. Effective teaching behaviors of rural family medicine preceptors. *CMAJ.* 1995;153(2):161–168

12. Hunter A, Desai S, Harrison R, Chan B. Medical student evaluation of the quality of hospitalist and nonhospitalist teaching faculty on inpatient medicine rotations. *Acad Med.* 2004;79(1):78–82

13. Dolmans DH, Wolfhagen IH, Essed GG, Scherpbier AJ, van der Vleuten CP. The impacts of supervision, patient mix, and numbers of students on the effectiveness of clinical rotations. *Acad Med.* 2002;77(4):332–335

14. Elnicki D, Kolarik R, Bardella I. Third-year medical students' perceptions of effective teaching behaviors in a multidisciplinary ambulatory clerkship. *Acad Med.* 2003;78(8):815–819

15. Masunaga H, Hitchcock MA. Residents' and faculty's beliefs about the ideal clinical teacher. *Fam Med.* 2010;42(2):116–120

16. Buchel TL, Edwards FD. Characteristics of effective clinical teachers. *Fam Med.* 2005;37(1):30–35

The views expressed in this article are those of the authors and do not necessarily represent those of the Uniformed Services University or the US Department of Defense.

FINANCIAL DISCLOSURE: *The authors have indicated they have no financial relationships relevant to this article to disclose.*

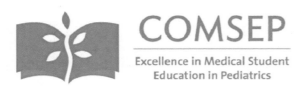
COMSEP
Excellence in Medical Student
Education in Pediatrics

AUTHORS: Susan L. Bannister, MD, MEd,[a] Hayley M. Wickenheiser, BKin, and David A. Keegan, MD[b]

Departments of [a]Paediatrics and [b]Family Medicine, University of Calgary, Alberta, Canada

Address correspondence to Susan L. Bannister, MD, MEd, Department of Paediatrics, Alberta Children's Hospital, 2888 Shaganappi Trail NW, Calgary AB, T3B 6A8, Canada. E-mail: susan.bannister@albertahealthservices.ca

Accepted for publication Nov 18, 2013

KEY WORDS
teamwork, leadership, interprofessionalism, medical education

Drs Bannister and Keegan conceptualized the article, and together with Ms Wickenheiser, they developed the framework described in the manuscript. Dr Bannister wrote the first draft of the manuscript. All authors contributed to the literature search, reviewed and revised the manuscript, and approved the final manuscript as submitted.

doi:10.1542/peds.2013-3734

Key Elements of Highly Effective Teams

The Council on Medical Student Education in Pediatrics (COMSEP) is an organization that values — and appreciates the benefits of — teams. COMSEP's best work comes as a result of highly effective teamwork.

A team is more than 1 person working together toward a common goal. Therefore, every physician is on multiple teams, ranging from a small team of himself or herself and a patient and family, to primary care medical home teams, to inpatient care teams with various levels of trainees and different professionals, to clinical and basic science research teams, to hospital boards, university committees, and organized community initiatives. Knowing the key elements of highly effective teams is relevant to every clinician, no matter where he or she practices.

In health care, team communication failures contribute to health care errors.[1] Effective teams decrease length of stay, result in fewer unanticipated admissions, improve coordination of care, decrease wait times, increase patient satisfaction, and improve health outcomes.[2]

The literature on teams is complex. A wide variety of conceptual frameworks[3] have been developed independently, and as a result, they are not aligned with each other.[4] In the health care literature specifically, a large number of team models have been proposed.[5–7]

In this article, we present a novel way to think about team effectiveness that is easy to remember and can be used to set your team up for success and resolve common barriers. Drawing on the business, sports, and interprofessional health care literature, we have identified 3 key elements: purpose, openness, and roles and skills (Table 1 summarizes the features of each of these elements). This framework can be applied in physicians' clinical, educational, and administrative roles to assist with team effectiveness.

KEY ELEMENTS OF HIGHLY EFFECTIVE TEAMS

Purpose

Having a common purpose that all team members can articulate is fundamental.[8] It could be "diagnosing what's go-ing on with Emily," "caring for our team of inpatients while completing the objectives of the rotation," or "efficiently managing resources in an outpatient clinic." Teams need to involve all members in purpose development; everyone should be able to articulate the team's purpose and be committed to it.[9] If team members have different understandings of what their common purpose is, friction, confusion, and a waste of resources and effort are inevitable, and it will be harder to get the team back on track.

An important challenge teams face occurs when the original purpose is superseded by a new, different purpose. Effective teams know shifts in purpose can occur. As a result, they check in regularly with both their members and external stakeholders to ensure that the purpose is still right. By checking in, teams determine whether they need to change their purpose or direction. For instance, in a clinical setting, the goal of

TABLE 1 Summary of Key Elements of Highly Effective Teams

Purpose	Openness	Roles and Skills
Clear	Excellent communication	Right people
Shared	Mutual respect	Right skills
Regular checking in	Safe environment	Awareness of each other's roles
Focus on "what's important now"	Leaderful	Necessary tools and resources
Celebrate successes	Engaged	are provided

a specific patient's care may change from diagnosis to cure, and later to optimizing the patient's quality of life; on a committee, a new external mandate may require the team to change its focus.

Deciding whether to change purpose can be challenging. According to former Notre Dame football coach Lou Holtz, a team has to concentrate on W.I.N.: "what's important now."[10] In this approach, a team openly discusses events, new information, and changing circumstances and asks, "What's important now?" This approach helps the team distinguish between things that should trigger a change in strategy and things that should be ignored or coped with. Effective teams ask themselves, "Does this need to be dealt with now?" (If yes, deal with it.) "Does this issue have the power to impede the team's progress?" (If yes, deal with it now.)[8]

As progress toward a goal is made, it is important to celebrate achievements, even small ones; it helps keep the focus on the main purpose and builds team identity and momentum.[8,11]

Openness

We think of openness as encompassing excellent communication (including the ability to say "I don't know"), mutual respect and promoting a "leaderful team."[7,9,12]

Poor team communication can result in incomplete or inaccurate information being exchanged, important issues not being resolved, and key members being excluded.[13] Closed-loop communication is 1 way to address these issues.[14] Originally used in the military and most frequently used in health care in code situations, it requires team members to confirm they have heard instructions correctly and enables all members to be aware of what is happening.[14]

An important predictor of a team's success is the team's pattern of communication

and the energy and engagement of the group outside team meetings.[15] Successful teams ensure that all members speak, and listen, and connect to one another. Pentland[15] emphasizes the importance of face-to-face communication, stating that 35% of the variation in a team's performance is related to the number of face-to-face exchanges between team members.

Members of an open team feel safe enough to speak up and raise additional or contrary opinions, or declare their areas of uncertainty and ignorance, with the knowledge that their concerns will be listened to carefully.[16,17] Leaders can promote an open team by posing thoughtful questions to the group and by declaring their own risk of making errors in judgment.[16]

To have a high degree of engagement, a team must function with mutual respect at all times. This can be difficult because of members' differing perspectives, arising from different backgrounds and group cultures.[7] However, different perspectives also enable a team to spot previously unrecognized opportunities and challenges; as a result, they should be sought out, shared, and respected.[16]

The culture of an open team naturally enables it to be "leaderful"[12] in that all members feel empowered to jointly share in leadership tasks, such as ensuring that viewpoints have been explored and difficult issues raised. A leaderful team can have more than 1 leader operating at a time, and they do so in a collective manner, striving for the common purpose.[12] Leaderful practice is collaborative; members operate in good faith and seek to ensure that all members are engaged.[12]

Changing a traditional leadership culture to a leaderful one is challenging. It takes time, an open culture, a leader who is willing to allow others to lead,

and team members who are willing to lead even when they do not feel comfortable.[12]

Roles and Skills

Teams that are purpose oriented and open still need 1 more element to be successful: they need to have the right people with the right skills. Team members need to know who is on the team and what they each contribute in terms of skills and knowledge.[18] Each team member must understand his or her role and those of others on the team.[9] Any tools or resources needed to enable team members to fulfill their roles must be provided.[18,19]

The team needs to be aware of any gaps between the skills present on the team and the skills needed to accomplish the purpose. This knowledge will directly drive additional training or the targeted recruitment of additional team members.

WHEN THINGS GO WRONG

Sometimes things do not work well. For instance, the team may not function well, the team may not have been set up for success, or external events may have derailed the team's progress. To find out what went wrong, a team should ask the following questions based on the 3 key elements described in this article:

● Do we have a clear purpose?

● Are we fostering an open environment?

● Do we have the necessary people with the necessary skills and resources on our team? Do they know their (and others') role?

There will always be challenges in a team environment; having a plan to respond to them is crucial.[8] Effective teams get back on track by exploring what went wrong and looking for the opportunities that lie within setbacks.[8,9]

CONCLUSIONS

All physicians are members of teams. The teams that have a clear, shared purpose, that are open and leaderful (including encouraging every member to contribute regardless of his or her status), and whose members have role awareness and the right skills are the ones that are set up for success.

REFERENCES

1. Sutcliffe KM, Lewton E, Rosenthal MM. Communication failures: an insidious contributor to medical mishaps. *Acad Med.* 2004;79(2):186–194

2. Mickan SM. Evaluating the effectiveness of health care teams. *Aust Health Rev.* 2005;29 (2):211–217

3. Salas E, Stagl K, Burke CS. 25 years of team effectiveness in organizations: research themes and emerging needs. In: Cooper CL, Robertson IT, eds. *International Review of Industrial and Organizational Psychology.* New York, NY: Wiley; 2004:47–91

4. Rousseau V, Aubé C, Savoie A. Teamwork behaviors: a review and an integration of frameworks. *Small Group Res.* 2006;37(5): 540–570

5. Lo L. *Teamwork and Communication in Healthcare: A Literature Review.* Edmonton, AB, Canada: Canadian Patient Safety Institute; 2001

6. Mickan S, Rodger S. Characteristics of effective teams: a literature review. *Aust Health Rev.* 2000;23(3):201–208

7. Mickan SM, Rodger SA. Effective health care teams: a model of six characteristics developed from shared perceptions. *J Interprof Care.* 2005;19(4):358–370

8. Wickenheiser H. *Gold Medal Diary: Inside the World's Greatest Sports Event.* Vancouver, BC, Canada: Greystone Books Ltd.; 2010

9. Benincasa R. *How Winning Works: 8 Essential Leadership Lessons From the Toughest Teams on Earth.* Don Mills, ON, Canada: Harlequin; 2012

10. Holtz L. *Winning Every Day.* New York, NY: Harper Business; 1998

11. Kouzes JM, Posner BZ. *The Leadership Challenge: How to Make Extraordinary Things Happen in Organizations.* 5th ed. San Francisco, CA: Jossey-Bass; 2012

12. Raelin JA. *The Leaderful Fieldbook: Strategies and Activities for Developing Leadership in Everyone.* Boston, MA: Davies-Black; 2010

13. Lingard L, Espin S, Whyte S, et al. Communication failures in the operating room: an observational classification of recurrent types and effects. *Qual Saf Health Care.* 2004;13(5):330–334

14. Burke CS, Salas E, Wilson-Donnelly K, Priest H. How to turn a team of experts into an expert medical team: guidance from the aviation and military communities. *Qual Saf Health Care.* 2004;13(1 suppl):i96–i104

15. Pentland A. The new science of building great teams: the chemistry of high-performing groups is no longer a mystery. *Harv Bus Rev.* 2012;3:61–70

16. Edmondson AC. Teamwork on the fly: how to master the new art of teaming. *Harv Bus Rev.* 2012;3:72–80

17. Gardner HK. Coming through when it matters most: how great teams do their best work under pressure. *Harv Bus Rev.* 2012;3: 83–91

18. Bohlman LG, Deal TE. *Re-framing Organizations: Artistry, Choice and Leadership.* 5th ed. San Francisco, CA: Jossey-Bass; 2012

19. Hertzberg F, Mausner B, Snyderman B. *The Motivation to Win.* 2nd ed. New York, NY: John Wiley & Sons; 1959

FINANCIAL DISCLOSURE: The authors have indicated they have no financial relationships relevant to this article to disclose.
FUNDING: No external funding.
POTENTIAL CONFLICT OF INTEREST: The authors have indicated they have no potential conflicts of interest relevant to this article to disclose.

How to "ENGAGE" Multilevel Learner Groups in the Clinical Setting

Patricia D. Quigley, MD, MME,[a] Nicholas M. Potisek, MD,[b] Michael A. Barone, MD, MPH[c]

In many clinical settings, multiple trainees work alongside a single preceptor. Not surprisingly, there is great variability in the knowledge and skills of medical students, residents, fellows, and other health professions trainees. In such settings, it can be challenging to engage the entire team while avoiding teaching that any particular trainee would perceive as too elementary or too complex. Thus, great clinical teachers employ strategies to develop different learners' clinical skills and independence. Unfortunately, not much information is available on this topic, and clinical teachers may only find effective teaching strategies for such multilevel learner (MLL) groups by trial and error.[1–4]

A quick assessment of learners' needs and educational levels forms the foundation of teaching MLLs. When joining an inpatient team or starting a day in the outpatient clinic, the great clinical teacher finds out who are the medical, physician assistant, nursing, or therapy students and who are the interns, senior residents, or fellows. Experienced preceptors seek opportunities to talk with learners one-to-one, ask about their interests, and work with them to develop 1 or 2 specific learning goals. Great teachers ask skillful questions to gain insight into each learner's unique experiences, knowledge base, and

adeptness with clinical reasoning.[5] The reporter-interpreter-manager-educator framework may provide a useful approach to assessing a learner's sophistication with clinical reasoning and patient care.[6]

In this article from the Council on Medical Students in Pediatrics series on great clinical teachers, we offer specific strategies for teaching learners who are at different levels. The ENGAGE mnemonic (Everyone teaches, Novel topics, Guide, Ascend the ladder, Groups within the group, Empower learners for autonomy) provides preceptors with a toolbox for engaging all levels of learners (Fig 1). Throughout this article, we provide examples for teaching through an illustrative case of a 4-year-old boy presenting with symptoms of Kawasaki disease (KD).

E: EVERYONE TEACHES

Great clinical teachers set the expectation that all learners will contribute to teaching, often relating opportunities for teaching to each learner's individualized learning goals.[7] The clinical teacher can guide learners to present succinct, clinically relevant teaching points that fill knowledge gaps for those on the team. Topics can be assigned or learners may volunteer insights from their own studying. Interprofessional staff offer unique perspectives, and

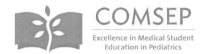

[a]Division of General Pediatrics, Johns Hopkins All Children's Hospital, St. Petersburg, Florida; [b]Department of Pediatrics, Wake Forest Baptist Medical Center, Winston-Salem, North Carolina; and [c]Department of Pediatrics, School of Medicine, Johns Hopkins University, Baltimore, Maryland

Dr Quigley conceptualized the ENGAGE mnemonic, drafted the initial manuscript, revised the manuscript, and developed Fig 1; Dr Potisek conceptualized the ENGAGE mnemonic, drafted portions of the initial manuscript, and revised subsequent versions; Dr Barone conceptualized the ENGAGE mnemonic and reviewed and revised the manuscript; and all authors approved the final manuscript as submitted and agree to be accountable for all aspects of the work.

DOI: https://doi.org/10.1542/peds.2017-2861

Accepted for publication Aug 23, 2017

Address correspondence to Patricia D. Quigley, MD, MME, Johns Hopkins All Children's Hospital, Office of Medical Education, 601 5th Ave S, Saint Petersburg, FL 33701. E-mail: patricia.quigley@jhmi.edu

PEDIATRICS (ISSN Numbers: Print, 0031-4005; Online, 1098-4275).

FINANCIAL DISCLOSURE: The authors have indicated they have no financial relationships relevant to this article to disclose.

FUNDING: No external funding.

POTENTIAL CONFLICT OF INTEREST: The authors have indicated they have no potential conflicts of interest to disclose.

To cite: Quigley PD, Potisek NM, Barone MA. How to "ENGAGE" Multilevel Learner Groups in the Clinical Setting. *Pediatrics.* 2017;140(5):e20172861

Step 1: Plan Consider Patients and Learning Opportunities	Step 2: Assess Assess Learners' Needs in the Clinical Setting	Step 3: Teach Select a Teaching Strategy (ENGAGE)
Identify level of medical complexity of the patients on the ward or clinic schedule Locate clinical guidelines, studies, and/or protocols that apply to the types of patients to be seen Identify challenging social, economic, or community factors that are likely to be relevant List work that needs to be done for the patients (H&P, literature review, follow up laboratory results)	Identify the individual learning goals of each learner Relate selected teaching topics to individual learning goals Plan according to individual and group knowledge gaps Identify the learners' future levels of autonomy (PA versus APRN versus general pediatrician versus orthopedic surgeon) Assess learners' levels of clinical reasoning: **Reporter:** able to gather data **Interpreter:** able to interpret data and assess patient **Manager:** able to manage treatment, negotiation, consults **Educator:** able to teach peers, patients, and families	**Everyone teaches:** all team members contribute to daily learning • Medical students and interns: Brief teaching reports • Senior residents and fellows: On-the-fly teaching • Interprofessional staff: Share their clinical perspectives • Family: clinical course of disease **Novel topics:** collectively review new guidelines, studies, and protocols • Assign pairs or groups to review guidelines appropriate to level **Guide:** explicitly role model humanism, professionalism, communication, or diagnostic bias • Reflect out loud • Demonstrate vulnerability • As a team, consider multiple perspectives about a patient • Role play difficult conversations **Ascend the ladder:** targeted questioning of each team member to build shared understanding • Question based on anticipated knowledge base of each learner • Ask the same question of each learner, starting with the most junior (e.g., What is your assessment of this patient?) **Groups within the group:** create pairs or trios to complete a task • Pairs to answer a clinical question and share findings • Pair medical students with residents to create coaching relationships • When possible, pair learners according to complementary skills or similar learning goals. **Empower learners for autonomy:** promote autonomy among all team members • Delegate duties appropriate to each learner's level of training • Encourage junior learners to lead discussions • Encourage team members to speak up with concerns

FIGURE 1

Steps to ENGAGE learners in MLL setting. APRN, advanced practice registered nurse; H&P, history and physical examination; PA, physician's assistant.

patients and family members can teach about their experiences with diagnosis, treatment, and advocacy.

In our example, the 4-year-old boy initially presents to clinic. The intern, interested in pediatric rheumatology, has never cared for a child with KD. The great clinical teacher, aware of the learner's interests and that this patient may have KD, asks the intern to evaluate the patient and review the diagnostic criteria with other learners. After the encounter, the students may teach features of incomplete KD. During the hospital admission, the inpatient team may ask pharmacy staff to teach about side effects of intravenous immunoglobulin (IVIg) and nursing staff to discuss monitoring parameters during IVIg administration. Families may provide

a narrative of the natural history of KD in their child.

N: NOVEL TOPICS

Clinical teachers can introduce recent publications, hospital protocols, clinical guidelines, and new understandings of disease mechanisms or treatments. By teaching novel topics, the clinical teacher models "keeping up to date" throughout one's career.

In our patient encounter, the teacher can compare new KD guidelines with previous versions. Junior learners could present the rationale for revisions or other aspects of the new guidelines keyed to their level of learning. During a time set aside for teaching, senior learners can analyze how the coexistence of KD and viral

infection can lead to diagnostic uncertainty.

G: GUIDE

Role modeling is a powerful teaching strategy for MLLs, particularly for harder-to-teach competencies such as professionalism and humanism. Clinical teachers might assume learners notice the way they interact with a patient, but learners, who are not primed to notice these actions, may miss them. Saying, "I said [this] to the patient because…" often helps learners notice and internalize the learning point.

For example, the clinical teacher could model family-centered care. When hearing a parent's concerns about the risks of IVIg treatment, the clinical teacher may take an extra moment to understand and address the parent's concern rather than quoting data on the effectiveness of IVIg. Afterward, the teacher can lead a reflective discussion of the encounter. The teacher could ask the medical student to identify the differing perspectives that emerged from the conversation, the interns to reflect on how the varied perspectives converge or conflict, and/or a senior resident to walk the team through ways to reassure the worried parent, all without compromising treatment.[7]

A: ASCEND THE LADDER

Questioning by ascending "up the ladder"[8] helps the clinical teacher target specific learning objectives for each team member. The teacher asks developmentally appropriate questions of each learner based on their needs. Initially, the teacher may ask students foundational questions, such as questions about disease pathophysiology. Building on this discussion, the clinical teacher may prompt a more experienced learner to address diagnostic and treatment options. To conclude the discussion, the most experienced learner may be asked to describe a higher-order concept, such as case synthesis.[5] Questioning requires special attention, and many recommendations for skillful questioning appear in a previous Council on Medical Students in Pediatrics article.[5]

In our example, the clinical teacher may ask a medical student to discuss the pharmacotherapy of KD, whereas an intern may be asked to review the rates of IVIg treatment failure. A senior resident could review treatment options available should IVIg and aspirin fail.

G: GROUPS WITHIN THE GROUP

Establishing small groups (pairs or trios) within the larger clinical team, with each group focusing on a task,

promotes collaboration, teamwork, and leadership. Pair a senior resident with a medical student to create a coaching dyad for feedback on history and physical examinations and documentation or to staff patients in clinic. During group teaching, generate discussion and build consensus. For example, when faced with clinical uncertainty, as in refractory KD, pair learners to debate treatment options. After a brief discussion, join pairs to make a group of 4 and so on until 2 groups remain to debate and recommend treatment.

E: EMPOWER LEARNERS FOR AUTONOMY

Physicians and other health care providers are expected to develop increasing autonomy in caring for patients. Opportunities for autonomy are more apparent for senior learners, although there are ways to encourage autonomy among junior learners. Delegate duties appropriate to each learner's level and skill set. For example, allow the intern in the clinic to call the inpatient team to admit the patient with KD while the senior resident coordinates bed placement. Ask junior learners to lead discussions. Remind them to speak up with concerns about patient care. Support senior learners leading rounds with and without an attending physician present.[9,10] Recognize that readiness for autonomy does not necessarily correlate with the learner's level in their program, and encourage learners to follow their individual trajectories.

CONCLUSIONS

ENGAGE strategies for MLLs apply to both inpatient and ambulatory settings and will enable the great clinical teacher to meet the needs of individual learners while ensuring that patients and families receive timely and excellent care. After incorporating these strategies, the

clinical teacher will find that any setting with learners at multiple levels can become a dynamic environment in which everyone learns.

ACKNOWLEDGMENTS

We thank Janice Hanson, PhD, and Robert Dudas, MD, for their thoughtful reviews of the manuscript. Dr Hanson also helped to conceptualize Figure 1.

ABBREVIATIONS

IVIg: intravenous immunoglobulin
KD: Kawasaki disease
MLL: multilevel learner

REFERENCES

1. Castiglioni A, Shewchuk RM, Willett LL, Heudebert GR, Centor RM. A pilot study using nominal group technique to assess residents' perceptions of successful attending rounds. *J Gen Intern Med.* 2008;23(7):1060–1065

2. Tariq M, Motiwala A, Ali SU, Riaz M, Awan S, Akhter J. The learners' perspective on internal medicine ward rounds: a cross-sectional study. *BMC Med Educ.* 2010;10:53

3. Stickrath C, Aagaard E, Anderson M. MiPLAN: a learner-centered model for bedside teaching in today's academic medical centers. *Acad Med.* 2013;88(3):322–327

4. Chen HC, Fogh S, Kobashi B, Teherani A, Ten Cate O, O'Sullivan P. An interview study of how clinical teachers develop skills to attend to different level learners. *Med Teach.* 2016;38(6):578–584

5. Long M, Blankenburg R, Butani L. Questioning as a teaching tool. *Pediatrics.* 2015;135(3):406–408

6. Pangaro L. A new vocabulary and other innovations for improving descriptive in-training evaluations. *Acad Med.* 1999;74(11):1203–1207

7. Lockspeiser T, Schmitter P, Lane J, Hanson J, Rosenberg A. A validated rubric for scoring learning goals. *MedEdPORTAL Publications*. 2013;9:9369

8. Certain LK, Guarino AJ, Greenwald JL. Effective multilevel teaching techniques on attending rounds: a pilot survey and systematic review of the literature. *Med Teach*. 2011;33(12):e644–e650

9. Seltz LB, Preloger E, Hanson JL, Lane L. Ward rounds with or without an attending physician: how interns learn most successfully. *Acad Pediatr*. 2016;16(7):638–644

10. Montacute T, Chan Teng V, Chen Yu G, Schillinger E, Lin S. Qualities of resident teachers valued by medical students. *Fam Med*. 2016;48(5):381–384

The Clinical COACH: How to Enable Your Learners to Own Their Learning

Susan L. Bannister, MD, MEd, FRCPC,[a,b] Theresa F. Wu, MD, MSc, FRCPC,[a,b] David A. Keegan, MD, CCFP(EM), FCFP[c]

The ultimate goal of medical education is for learners to become competent physicians who identify learning needs from patient encounters, from system issues, and even from mistakes, and proactively develop educational plans to fill those needs. With this article, we continue the Council on Medical Student Education in Pediatrics series about the skills and strategies of great clinical teachers by illuminating the coaching role teachers can play in developing lifelong learners.

Clinical teachers supervise clinical learners as they jointly provide medical care to patients. A key role is to provide feedback to learners; however, this can be a struggle because most clinical teachers have received little instruction in giving feedback.[1] Clinical teachers also may believe providing constructive feedback is often done in vain, because of a lack of resources to help the learner improve.[1] Teachers may worry about damaging their relationship with learners or about hurting the learners' self-esteem.[2] Learners contribute to the challenges within this teacher-learner feedback relationship, because they often avoid asking for feedback for fear it will be critical and may become defensive when offered corrective feedback, particularly if they worry about feedback hurting their grades.[3]

Feedback and coaching are different. The focus of "feedback" is often on the tasks that teachers do (how to deliver feedback, when to have such conversations, etc) to direct the construction of a learning plan. Often, feedback is given about something decided on by the teacher rather than that requested by the learner. There are other ways to help students develop. Advising and mentoring are also directed by the preceptor, and his or her role is to provide advice or guidance over a short- or long-term period, respectively. On the other hand, the key features of "coaching" are that the coach encourages the learner to reflect, gain insight, address and solve problems, and take responsibility for his or her own learning and growth.[4,5]

Whitmore's[6] general coaching model, not specific to medical education, describes the following 4 steps for effective coaching: help the learner articulate Goals, reflect on Reality or current abilities, describe Options for learning, and decide on a plan (What they want to do/are going to do). The resulting acronym "GROW" is meant as a general coaching framework for helping someone get to an "inspirational" or "stretch" goal over a substantial period of time.[6] The R2C2 model[7] describes 4 phases for assessment discussions with medical learners: (1) develop Rapport and relationship, (2) explore the trainee's Reactions to the feedback, (3) assist in understanding Content of feedback, and (4) Coach to

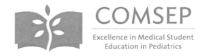

Departments of *Paediatrics and *Family Medicine, Cumming School of Medicine, University of Calgary, Calgary, Alberta, Canada; and *Alberta Children's Hospital, Calgary, Alberta, Canada

Dr Bannister conceptualized the Clinical COACH feedback model, drafted the initial manuscript, and reviewed and revised the manuscript; Dr Wu conceptualized the Clinical COACH feedback model and critically reviewed and revised the manuscript; Dr Keegan conceptualized the Clinical COACH feedback model, critically reviewed and revised the manuscript for important intellectual content, and oversaw the design of the model; and all authors approved the final manuscript as submitted and agree to be accountable for all aspects of the work.

DOI: https://doi.org/10.1542/peds.2018-2601

Accepted for publication Aug 20, 2018

Address correspondence to Susan L. Bannister, MD, MEd, FRCPC, Department of Paediatrics, University of Calgary, Alberta Children's Hospital, 2888 Shaganappi Trail NW, Calgary, AB, Canada T3B 6A8. E-mail: susan.bannister@ahs.ca

PEDIATRICS (ISSN Numbers: Print, 0031-4005; Online, 1098-4275).

FINANCIAL DISCLOSURE: The authors have indicated they have no financial relationships relevant to this article to disclose.

FUNDING: No external funding.

POTENTIAL CONFLICT OF INTEREST: The authors have indicated they have no potential conflicts of interest to disclose.

To cite: Bannister SL, Wu TF, Keegan DA. The Clinical COACH: How to Enable Your Learners to Own Their Learning. *Pediatrics.* ;142(5):e20182601

TABLE 1 The Clinical COACH Model

Step	Purpose	Potential Questions and Statements
Contract for the learning relationship	The learning goals of the learner are shared and explored. The teacher and learner come to an agreement on coaching as the guiding model for the learning relationship, with a clear understanding of each other's roles.	"My role is to be your coach. Do you know how coaching is different from giving feedback?" "My job is to ask lots of questions – to help you identify your learning needs." "What do you think about this coaching model of preceptoring?" "Is there anything you need or need to know to help you thrive in this model?" "What do you see as your role in a coaching relationship?" "Are we good to go?"
Optimize the learning environment to be able to recognize and capture learning moments	Developing the clinical environment to position the teacher at the right place, at the right time, and with the right information is key to identifying moments for coaching. Directly observing portions of the learner's patient interactions, reviewing the learner's clinical notes in real time, and getting feedback from patients, family, and clinical staff are some examples of optimization.	"I'd like to join you when you discuss this issue with the patient and family." "Please try and prioritize the completion of your clinical notes so I can review them as the day proceeds." A question that can be addressed to a patient or family member is as follows: "Can you give me any insight on areas where [the learner] is strong, and where [the learner] may need to improve?"

Act to provide coaching in the moment	When the teacher becomes aware of an area for learner growth, the teacher engages with the learner to ensure the learner (1) is aware and understands the performance issue, (2) has an appropriate performance goal for improvement, and (3) has a good plan on how to develop any missing skills or knowledge.	(1) Awareness (examples are provided with increasing levels of direction)
		   "What did you think about the last patient encounter?"
		   "Did you notice the patient's mother seemed quite reluctant to get the test?"
		   "What might be some reasons why this mother would be reluctant?"
		(2) Goal
		   "What would you say is your responsibility as a clinician when you are putting together a care plan?"
		   "Think of really great doctors you have worked with. How do they work with patients and families to develop care plans?"
		   "Are you aware of any frameworks that physicians use with patients and families to create care plans that meet everyone's needs?"
		(3) Plan
		   "Can you share how you will handle this kind of conversation the next time?"
		   "Have you developed a plan to hold these kinds of conversations?"
		   "Do you need my help in identifying a good resource to learn from?"

Check in (1) on learner plans and outcomes and (2) the coaching relationship	It is important as a coach to check in with the learner to ensure the identified plans have been undertaken, with new learning being applied. Additionally, it is important to check in on the coaching relationship and make any required modifications.	Learner plans
		   "Can you share with me any key things you learned?"
		   "Have you been able to apply what you learned? How is it going?"
		   "Do you think you've got this part solved? Or do you think you have more room to grow?"
		Coaching relationship
		   "How is this coaching process working for you?"
		   "Are the questions I ask you helpful?"
		   "Am I doing too much or too little coaching?"

identify performance or knowledge gaps, then set goals and plans.[7] The authors of the R2C2 model note a key limitation is the time required to conduct an R2C2 session, which may limit its use in some circumstances in busy clinical settings.[7]

HOW TO COACH IN A BUSY CLINICAL PRACTICE

Adding coaching sessions into a clinical teacher's schedule may seem daunting. Coachable moments can be identified and efficiently acted on, however, during clinical encounters. We have drawn from key literature about orientation,[8] learning environments,[9] coaching,[4–7] and closed-loop communication[10] to create a 4-step model for coaching in the moment called the Clinical COACH. The key actions for each step of this model (contact, optimize, act, check-in) make up the mnemonic COACH. Table 1 describes each of the 4 steps of this model, along with potential sentences and questions appropriate for teachers to use. Figure 1 provides a quick overview of the Clinical COACH model.

Step 1: Contract

Orienting learners to a clinical environment assists in the creation of good clinical learning environments.[8] During orientation, the teacher works with the learner to create a shared understanding of their coaching

The Clinical COACH
Pediatrics Quick Card

1. Contract
- part of orientation
- explore learner's goals
- establish agreement on what each person's role is
- eg "My job is to ask questions to help you identify your areas for growth. Is this okay?"

2. Optimize
- set things up to be in the right places at the right times to observe and coach
- eg extra stools in rooms, whiteboards, read notes

3. Act
(a) Is the learner aware of the performance issue?
(b) Does the learner have an appropriate goal for their improvement?
(c) Does the learner have a solid plan for getting to their goal?

4. Check-in
- Is the learner implementing the plans? How are the outcomes?
- How is the relationship working? Does something need to change?

Based on Bannister SL, Wu TF, Keegan DA. The Clinical COACH: How to enable your learners to own their learning. *Pediatrics.* 2018;142(5): e20182601.

FIGURE 1
The Clinical COACH Quick Card (may be cut out and folded into a handy reminder card).

relationship. This conversation includes sharing and exploring the learner's goals and the roles each will have as coach and learner.

Step 2: Optimize

The teacher explores and implements ways to optimize his or her ability to coach, by being in the right places at the right times to identify moments when coaching can be helpful. Examples include having an extra stool in the examination room to facilitate in-room observation, extra paper or a white board readily available to provide visual aids, or extra examination equipment available for demonstration and practice. The learner should be empowered to ask the teacher to observe activities around which they desire coaching. The teacher should also seek out feedback from patients, families, and others in the health care environment, to identify potential areas for coaching.

Step 3: Act

The teacher coaches his or her learner in the moment around a recently observed action or behavior.

The key roles of the coach in this phase are to see if the learner is (1) aware of the performance issue, (2) has an appropriate goal for performance improvement, and (3) has a good plan to reach that goal. The teacher may help the learner gain awareness by encouraging self-reflection. Some examples could include asking, "I noticed you struggled during the difficult conversation. How did you feel your encounter with the parent went?" Once the learner has reflected and gained awareness of the performance issue, teachers can help the learner identify a goal. For example, "How skilled do you think you should be in holding goals of care conversations?" Once the performance goal has been identified, the teacher will coach the learner to create a plan to achieve it. "Have you thought of ways to develop the skills needed for you to hold goals of care conversations?"

Step 4: Check-in

Teachers check in at the end of each in-the-moment coaching session to ensure the learner has understood

the feedback and continues to be receptive to further coaching. Ideally, a coaching relationship will be longitudinal, and teachers should check in intermittently to ensure the relationship is going well. The teacher can invite suggestions from the learner on how to improve the relationship by asking, "How can we make our coaching relationship better?" Additionally, teachers in the check-in phase can reflect on their own role in the relationship. Questions such as "How am I doing?," "What can I change for future learners?," and "Do I need to alter the physical layout of the clinical space?" can guide self-reflection.

CONCLUSIONS

Effective coaching has the potential to enable learners to increase their clinical skills and lifelong learning strategies. When done well, coaching can help learners to reflect, gain insight, address and solve problems, and take responsibility for their own learning, which are skills that are not necessarily nurtured in traditional feedback models. With competency-based medical education emerging as an important model for physician training, clinical teachers will need to equip themselves with tools to foster learner-driven education. The Clinical COACH model can help great clinical teachers to succeed in accomplishing this.

ABBREVIATION

COACH: contact, optimize, act, check-in

REFERENCES

1. Dudek NL, Marks MB, Regehr G. Failure to fail: the perspectives of clinical supervisors. *Acad Med.* 2005;80(suppl 10):S84–S87

2. Henderson P, Ferguson-Smith AC, Johnson MH. Developing essential professional skills: a framework for

teaching and learning about feedback. *BMC Med Educ.* 2005;5(1):11

3. Hargreaves DH, Southworth GW, Stanley P, Ward SJ. *On-the-Job Training for Physicians.* London, United Kingdom: Royal Society of Medicine Press; 1997

4. Lovell B. What do we know about coaching in medical education? A literature review. *Med Educ.* 2018;52(4):376–390

5. Marcdante K, Simpson D. Choosing when to advise, coach, or mentor. *J Grad Med Educ.* 2018;10(2):227–228

6. Whitmore J. *Coaching for Performance: The Principles and Practice of Coaching and Leadership.* 5th ed. London, United Kingdom: Nicholas Brealey Publishing; 2017

7. Sargeant J, Lockyer J, Mann K, et al. Facilitated reflective performance feedback: developing an evidence- and theory-based model that builds relationship, explores reactions and content, and coaches for performance change (R2C2). *Acad Med.* 2015;90(12):1698–1706

8. Raszka WV Jr, Maloney CG, Hanson JL. Getting off to a good start: discussing goals and expectations with medical students. *Pediatrics.* 2010;126(2):193–195

9. Bannister SL, Hanson JL, Maloney CG, Dudas RA. Practical framework for fostering a positive learning environment. *Pediatrics.* 2015;136(1):6–9

10. Burke CS, Salas E, Wilson-Donnelly K, Priest H. How to turn a team of experts into an expert medical team: guidance from the aviation and military communities. *Qual Saf Health Care.* 2004;13(suppl 1): i96–i104

To Trust or Not to Trust? An Introduction to Entrustable Professional Activities

Janice L. Hanson, PhD, EdS,[a] Susan L. Bannister, MD, MEd[b]

As clinical teachers, we look for ways to inspire medical students to reach for excellence in their practice of medicine. Entrustable professional activities, or EPAs, can help us do just this. This article, next in the Council on Medical Student Education in Pediatrics series on clinical teaching, provides an introduction to EPAs. Clinical teachers have always made decisions about which tasks to entrust to medical students and EPAs bring that important experience and judgment into a framework that organizes students' learning. EPAs have been conceptualized and written for residents, fellows, physician assistants, and, more recently, medical students.

WHAT ARE ENTRUSTABLE PROFESSIONAL ACTIVITIES?

Entrustable professional activities (EPAs) provide a framework for describing what medical students are expected to be able to do before graduation from medical school. They break down the work of a doctor into tasks, such as taking a history, forming a differential diagnosis, or recognizing a sick patient and initiating treatment. The word "entrustable" is part of this framework because most physicians, when working with a learner, have asked themselves, consciously or unconsciously, "Do

I trust this learner to do that?" And, only if the answer is "yes" do they allow the learner to do the task. So, although EPAs sound new (and potentially confusing), they are built on a foundation that physicians have intuitively used. After working with a student, for instance, and watching him or her conduct histories and physical examinations, a physician will decide whether to trust the student to conduct future histories and physical examinations on his or her own. This decision will be based on several factors, including the accuracy of the information the student has provided in the past, how well the student recognizes his or her limitations, the complexity of the patient, the circumstances of the family, the nature of the task, and time constraints.[1] It really all comes down to whether the physician can affirmatively answer the question, "Do I trust the learner to do this?"

EPAs help the clinician make this everyday judgment about whether to trust a student with a specific task by stating the task explicitly.[2,3] A group of medical educators from across the United States and Canada has agreed on a set of 13 "core EPAs" (see Table 1) that all medical students should be entrusted to do by the time they graduate from medical school, with a supervisor nearby to help when needed.[4] These core EPAs include key aspects of

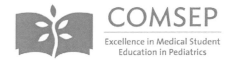

[a]Department of Pediatrics, University of Colorado School of Medicine, Aurora, Colorado; and [b]Department of Pediatrics, University of Calgary, Calgary, Alberta, Canada

Both authors contributed to the conceptualization of this article, drafting of the article, and revising it critically for important intellectual content, and approved the final version and agree to be accountable for all aspects of the work, including accuracy and integrity of all parts of the article.

DOI: 10.1542/peds.2016-2373

Accepted for publication Jul 19, 2016

Address correspondence to Janice Hanson, PhD, EdS, Department of Pediatrics, University of Colorado School of Medicine, 13123 E. 16th Ave, B-158, Aurora CO 80045. E-mail: janice.hanson@childrenscolorado.org

PEDIATRICS (ISSN Numbers: Print, 0031-4005; Online, 1098-4275).

FINANCIAL DISCLOSURE: The authors have indicated they have no financial relationships relevant to this article to disclose.

FUNDING: No external funding.

POTENTIAL CONFLICT OF INTEREST: The authors have indicated they have no potential conflicts of interest to disclose.

To cite: Hanson JL and Bannister SL. To Trust or Not to Trust? An Introduction to Entrustable Professional Activities. *Pediatrics.* 2016;138(5):e20162373

patient care and key components of working in a system of care.

ENTRUSTMENT AND SUPERVISION

"Entrustment" is assessed by deciding how much supervision a student needs to perform a particular professional activity when caring for patients. When an aspect of work is new for a student, the clinician may want the student to observe before practicing on his or her own. When students begin to practice on their own, the clinical teacher decides how much supervision they need. The clinician may stay in the room, watching everything they do. As they gain competence, they are trusted to practice with a clinician nearby who later double-checks what the student has done; then, after further practice and teaching, the clinician may double-check only key findings. The amount of supervision needed defines the level of entrustment.[10]

HOW ARE ENTRUSTMENT DECISIONS MADE?

How does a physician decide to trust a medical student to do something? This decision is often informed by many factors, such as the patient's acuity, the nature of the task, and the skill of the student. The following 5 factors describe the things that influence a physician's decision to trust a resident with a task. Physicians most likely consider many of the same things when deciding if a student can be trusted to perform a task.[11]

- The learner. Are they reliable? Truthful? Aware of their own limitations? What has been observed about their skill and competence?[12]

- The supervisor. The clinical teacher's own temperament and experience as a preceptor plays a role. Some teachers find it easy to trust each new student, unless the student does something that makes the clinician wary, whereas others

wait for each student to prove his or her trustworthiness in each new situation.

- The context. The clinical environment influences entrustment decisions, too. In a fast-paced clinical environment with few resources and many competing tasks, a student may be allowed less independence than in a less-intense setting.

- The task. The complexity of the patient's needs affects the level of supervision a student will need. Does the patient have a complex or unusual diagnosis, a complicated social situation, or many interrelated needs? Or does the patient have an urgent need? If so, a learner may need more supervision than he or she would if the learner was seeing a patient with a common, simple, single issue, or a patient with a common chronic condition that is well-managed.[1]

- The relationship between the learner and the supervisor. The relationship between the student and the clinical teacher also influences decisions about trust and supervision. Some learners spend only a few hours or days with a teacher, whereas other teachers and learners work together for several weeks or even longer. If they have developed shared expectations in the context of a working relationship, this can help to facilitate trust.

TEACHING AND ASSESSMENT BASED ON EPAS

Table 1 lists each of the 13 core EPAs[4] and provides examples from our experience of how to teach and assess each of these in a busy clinical setting.

What might a physician be asked to write on a form that uses EPAs to assess medical students? Instead of deciding if a student passes or fails

or "meets expectations" (which is often an abstract concept), a clinical teacher will be asked to make a decision that has clinical meaning; that is, can the student be entrusted or not to perform a certain task. The teacher will document what a student can do based on observations, direct supervision, feedback, and teaching. Teachers will be asked to justify their decisions with written examples of what the student did or did not do and how the student responded to feedback and progressed during the clinical experience.

The observations and assessments that the clinical teacher makes about a student become evidence of the student's progress. The teacher gathers evidence by observing the student in clinical encounters, coaching the student around presentations, and asking for the student's self-reflection after clinical encounters. The teacher provides evidence to the clerkship director by writing short examples of the student's performance that explain the teacher's judgment[13] and by choosing from a list of options that state how much supervision was needed. Although making judgments about students is a familiar task for many preceptors, it is often something that is done intuitively, without deliberate decision-making. Making these judgments deliberate and explicit provides the evidence that the clerkship director needs to reach conclusions about how the student has performed during the clerkship and also provides clear feedback for the student to guide efforts to improve.

CONCLUSIONS

EPAs provide a framework for describing the work that doctors do and the skills that medical students must acquire before graduation from medical school. This framework assists medical students because it clearly outlines what is expected, it allows students to focus on specific skills, and it demonstrates that one

TABLE 1 Ways to Teach and Assess EPAs

EPA[4]	Ways to Teach	Ways to Assess: Is This Student Entrustable?
EPA 1: Gather a history and perform a physical examination	• Ask student to observe you performing parts of a physical examination • Ask student to observe you asking questions • Direct student to open-access resources for taking a history and performing a physical examination, such as the Council on Medical Student Education in Pediatrics physical examination video[5] • Ask student to take patient's vital signs and conduct all or part of the physical examination (and then double-check) • Role play taking history with student	• Ask "What are the most important questions for this patient today? Why?" • Watch student perform components of the history and physical examination or confirm findings that were not observed • Ask "What are the most critical things to examine on this patient today? Why?" • Ask "What findings on physical examination rule in and rule out the working diagnosis?" • Ask patient and family if student asked questions in a logical, nonjudgmental, empathetic way • Ask patient and family if student examined patient in a way that promoted the patient's comfort • Ask patient and family if the student explained what he or she was doing
EPA 2: Prioritize a differential diagnosis following a clinical encounter	• Explain why you think a patient has a particular diagnosis • Explain what features on history and physical examination make that diagnosis most likely • Explain which other diagnoses need to be considered and relate them to features on the history and physical examination	• Ask student what the most likely diagnosis is and what features on history and physical examination led him or her to make that conclusion • Ask student what the alternate diagnoses are and what features on history and physical examination make those important to consider
EPA 3: Recommend and interpret common diagnostic and screening tests	• Explain why you are ordering tests • Explain how you are interpreting tests • Role model how to communicate effectively with patients and families and other members of the health care team about diagnostic and screening tests	• Ask student to interpret results from diagnostic tests • Ask students to explain how their approach to the patient would change if the test results were different • Ask student to explain the utility of the test • Ask student to explain how the test will be done and what the results may mean to a family
EPA 4: Enter and discuss orders and prescriptions	• Explain how to write orders • Detail the key components of a prescription • Let the student watch you document orders and prescriptions • Direct the student to a resource about how to write orders and prescriptions[6]	• Observe student explaining test results to a family • Review orders that student has documented • Review prescription that student has documented • Ask student to modify order and prescriptions for different clinical scenarios (eg, write on blank paper; vary the age, weight of patient, severity of illness, allergy history)
EPA 5: Document a clinical encounter in the patient record	• Provide a framework of what should be included in each of the following types of notes: admission note, progress note, procedure note, multidisciplinary meeting note, on-call note, discharge note	• Ask student to write admission note, progress note, procedure note, on-call note, multidisciplinary meeting note, discharge note in chart (if the student is not allowed to write in the chart, have the student write each of these notes for each patient on paper that is subsequently shredded) • Review the note for clarity, completeness, and documented understanding of the patient's issues and plans
EPA 6: Provide an oral presentation of a clinical encounter	• Provide a framework of what should be included in an effective oral presentation[7] • Ask the student to listen to one of your presentations (and see how well you followed the framework)	• Observe the student presenting a case on rounds or after a clinical encounter • Provide detailed, specific, feedback
EPA 7: Form clinical questions and retrieve evidence to advance patient care	• Model asking clinical questions and finding answers in the medical literature • Direct the student to resources at the university library	• Ask the student to form a clinical question about one of his or her patients • Ask the student to review the medical literature to answer that question • Review the student's search strategy and conclusions
EPA 8: Give or receive a patient handover to transition care responsibility	• Provide a framework of what should be included in handover (such as IPASS)[8] • Demonstrate how to effectively hand over a patient	• Watch the student give a patient handover • Do a "mock" handover; ask the student to present a short handover presentation to you • Assess the handover with an IPASS rating form • Ask "What does the next team need to know about this patient? What problems might evolve for this patient in the next 12 hours? How would you like the next team to manage those?"
EPA 9: Collaborate as a member of an interprofessional team	• If there are students from other professions (nursing students, pharmacy students, respiratory therapy students) at your site, consider arranging an interprofessional teaching session • Explain why you are engaging in an interprofessional team to provide patient care • Role model excellent and respectful communication	• Ask nurses and allied health personnel for feedback about the student • Ask student to document an interdisciplinary meeting • Observe student interacting with members of interprofessional team • Ask student what the role of each member of the team is and what skills each person brings • Ask student to consult with an interprofessional team member (eg, pharmacist, therapist, lactation consultant, nurse) to gather specific insights/information about a patient

TABLE 1 Continued

EPA[4]	Ways to Teach	Ways to Assess: Is This Student Entrustable?
EPA 10: Recognize a patient requiring urgent or emergent care and initiate evaluation and management	• Have student take Neonatal Resuscitation Program, Pediatric Advanced Life Support courses • Explain what it is about a particular patient that makes you know the patient is sick (eg, vitals, appearance)	• Ask student, "Is this patient sick or not sick? How do you know?" • Ask the student what the priorities are in management • Observe the student in a real or simulated scenario dealing with a sick patient
EPA 11: Obtain informed consent for tests and/or procedures	• Provide a framework of what should be included in such conversations[9] • Ask the student to observe you obtaining informed consent	• Observe the student obtaining consent • Ask the student about the risks and benefits of tests and procedures • Role play with the student
EPA 12: Perform general procedures of a physician (eg, basic cardiopulmonary resuscitation, bag and mask ventilation, venipuncture, inserting an intravenous line)	• Allow student to observe you perform procedures • Think out loud while demonstrating a procedure to explain the steps, the equipment, the indications and contraindications for the procedure • Use models for student to practice technical skills	• Observe the student perform the procedure on a model • Ask the student how the procedure would be performed differently for different patients ("What would you do differently if this patient was 1 week old? 3 years old? 15 years old? If the patient's weight was different? If the patient was acutely unwell?")
EPA 13: Identify system failures and contribute to a culture of safety and improvement	• Overtly discuss how you deal with system errors • Ask interprofessional team members to identify system errors they see and discuss them with the student • Encourage student to attend, and reflect on, morbidity and mortality–type conference	• Ask the student to identify a system failure • Observe the student disclosing an adverse outcome (to a patient and family or to yourself as part of a role play)

IPASS, Illness severity, Patient summary, Action list, Situation awareness and contingency planning, Synthesis by receiver.

can be doing well in one area and still have room to grow in another. Also, this framework can assist practicing physicians in teaching because it details what medical students need to be able to do. Instead of helping someone become a "good doctor," clinical teachers can focus their teaching, supervision, and feedback on helping students attain very specific skills, which will, ultimately, help their students become fine physicians.

ACKNOWLEDGMENTS

The authors thank William V. Razska, Jr, MD, and Meghan Trietz, MD, for their thoughtful reviews of this manuscript.

ABBREVIATION

EPAs: entrustable professional activities

REFERENCES

1. Ten Cate O, Hart D, Ankel F, et al; International Competency-Based Medical Education Collaborators. Entrustment decision making in clinical training. *Acad Med.* 2016;91(2):191–198

2. Ten Cate O. Entrustability of professional activities and competency-based training. *Med Educ.* 2005;39(12):1176–1177

3. Ten Cate O. Nuts and bolts of entrustable professional activities. *J Grad Med Educ.* 2013;5(1):157–158

4. Englander R, Aschenbrener CA, Call SA, et al; Association of American Medical Colleges. Core Entrustable Professional Acitivites for Entering Residency: Faculty and Learners' Guide. Available at: https://members.aamc.org/eweb/upload/Core EPA Faculty and Learner Guide.pdf

5. Council on Medical Student Education in Pediatrics (COMSEP). Multimedia Teaching Resources. 2016; includes video on the pediatric physical examination. Available at: https://www.comsep.org/educationalresources/multimediateachingtools.cfm. Accessed June 8, 2016

6. Ekong M, Frazier J, Oholendt K. How to write prescriptions. *MedEdPORTAL Publications.* 2014;10:9982

7. Bannister SL, Hanson JL, Maloney CG, Raszka WV Jr. Using the student case presentation to enhance diagnostic reasoning. *Pediatrics.* 2011;128(2):211–213

8. Starmer AJ, Spector ND, Srivastava R, Allen AD, Landrigan CP, Sectish TC; I-PASS Study Group. I-pass, a mnemonic to standardize verbal handoffs. *Pediatrics.* 2012;129(2):201–204

9. Fleisher L, Raivitch S, Miller SM, et al. A practical guide to informed consent. Available at: www.templehealth.org/ICTOOLKIT/html/ictoolkitpage20.html. Accessed June 8, 2016

10. Chen HC, McNamara M, Teherani A, Cate OT, O'Sullivan P. Developing entrustable professional activities for entry into clerkship. *Acad Med.* 2016;91(2):247–255

11. Hauer KE, Ten Cate O, Boscardin C, Irby DM, Iobst W, O'Sullivan PS. Understanding trust as an essential element of trainee supervision and learning in the workplace. *Adv Health Sci Educ Theory Pract.* 2014;19(3):435–456

12. Kennedy TJ, Regehr G, Baker GR, Lingard L. Point-of-care assessment of medical trainee competence for independent clinical work. *Acad Med.* 2008;83(suppl 10):S89–S92

13. Holmes AV, Peltier CB, Hanson JL, Lopreiato JO. Writing medical student and resident performance evaluations: beyond "performed as expected." *Pediatrics.* 2014;133(5):766–768

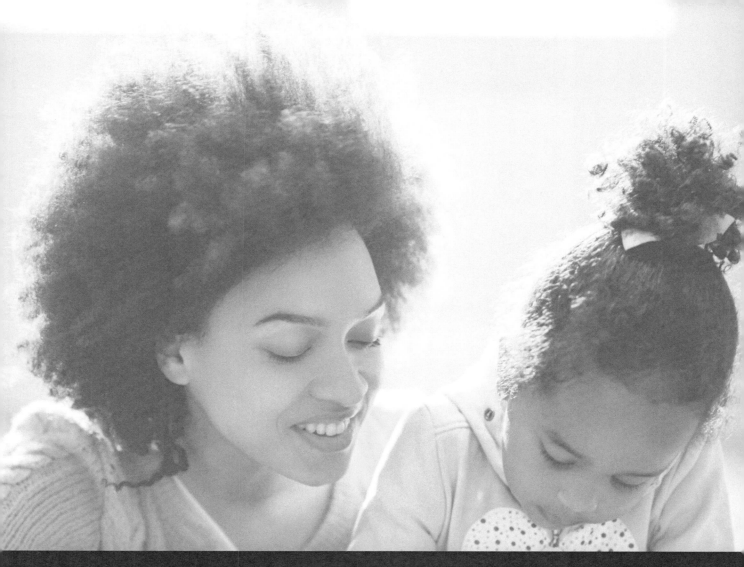

Chapter 3: Teaching Techniques

Chapter 3

Teaching Techniques: Incorporating Learning into a Busy Clinical Practice

By Robert A Dudas, MD
Associate Professor, Johns Hopkins University School of Medicine

Clinical teaching lies at the heart of medical education. For many pediatricians, the opportunity to teach future physicians brings tremendous personal and professional satisfaction. It is not easy, though. Competing demands and time pressures abound, while rewards and recognitions for teaching are often poor.[1] Additionally, many clinicians have not been taught how to teach well and are reliant upon their prior experiences as students themselves. As a result, they may overemphasize rote facts or underemphasize the importance of a positive learning environment.[1] As medical education continues to evolve into a specialized discipline, techniques, skills, and tools are being identified to assist teachers in maximizing the teaching and learning opportunities in the clinical setting.

This evolution has occurred slowly, but steadily. It was more than a century ago that Sir William Osler helped revolutionize both the delivery and teaching of medicine in North America. Importantly, he considered his advocacy for medical student training his most important career achievement.[2] Osler brought third-year students to outpatient clinics and fourth-year students to the wards at a time when most of medical education was lecture based.[2] He asserted that "...the natural method of teaching the student begins with the patient, continues with the patient, and ends his studies with the patient, using books and lectures as tools as means to an end."[3] He fostered a supportive learning environment with the hope that it would assist in creating physicians of high character. This included cultivating compassion toward patients by asking students to "care more particularly for the individual patient than for the special features of the disease."[4] These principles remain just as relevant today, as we see in the following collection of articles that seek to bring out the "inner Osler" of clinically busy pediatricians.

Indeed, the first article by Rideout et al encourages teachers to transition away from traditional lectures in which there tends to be a 1-way flow of information. The authors advocate for an "active learning" format that fosters lifelong learning by keeping things "short, active, and relevant" while maintaining the focus on patients.[5] Successive articles offer advice on how to pose good questions,[6] how to be more explicit when role modelling in a busy clinical environment,[7] and how to leverage mistakes as teaching opportunities.[8]

The subsequent articles ask pediatricians to "think out loud" to help students develop their clinical reasoning skills[9] as they transition from strict adherence to templates for the history and physical examination to a more advanced, nuanced, and hypothesis-driven approach.[10]

The article by Nagappan et al suggests that family-centered care provides an ideal framework to learn to "care more particularly for the individual patient" by demonstrating shared decision making while focusing on humanism and communication skills.[11] And in the last contribution, Dr Potisek shows a way to help students connect the dots between medical literature and patient care to help them learn to make evidence-based decisions.[12]

In the grand tradition of Sir William Osler, this collection of articles provides clinical teachers with strategies to teach and to foster student-centered active learning grounded in patient care.

References

1. Spencer J. Learning and teaching in the clinical environment. *BMJ*. 2003;326(7389):591–594. doi:10.1136/bmj.326.7389.591.
2. Bliss, Michael. *William Osler: A life in medicine*. New York: Oxford University Press, 1999. Print.
3. Osler W (Sir) Aequanimitas. 1945. The Blakiston Company, Philadelphia.
4. Charles S. Bryan (1999) Caring Carefully: Sir William Osier on the Issue of Competence vs Compassion in Medicine, Baylor University Medical Center Proceedings, 12:4,277-284, DOI: 10.1080/08998280.1999.11930198.
5. Rideout M, Held M, Holmes AV. The Didactic Makeover: Keep it Short, Active, Relevant. *Pediatrics*. 2016;138(1):e20160751. doi:10.1542/peds.2016-0751.
6. Long M, Blankenburg R, Butani L. Questioning as a teaching tool. *Pediatrics*. 2015;135(3):406–408. doi:10.1542/peds.2014-3285.
7. Potisek NM, Fromme B, Ryan MS. Transform Role Modeling Into SUPERmodeling. *Pediatrics*. 2019;144(5):e20192624. doi:10.1542/peds.2019-2624.
8. Beck JB, McGrath C, Toncray K, Rooholamini SN. Failure Is an Option: Using Errors as Teaching Opportunities. *Pediatrics*. 2018;141(3):e20174222. doi:10.1542/peds.2017-4222.
9. Bannister SL, Hanson JL, Maloney CG, Dudas RA. Just Do It: Incorporating Bedside Teaching Into Every Patient Encounter. *Pediatrics*. 2018;142(1):e20181238. doi:10.1542/peds.2018-1238.
10. Balighian E, Barone MA. Getting Physical: The Hypothesis Driven Physical Exam. *Pediatrics*. 2016;137(3):e20154511. doi:10.1542/peds.2015-4511.
11. Nagappan S, Hartsell A, Chandler N. Teaching in a family-centered care model: the exam room as the classroom. *Pediatrics*. 2013;131(5):836–838. doi:10.1542/peds.2013-0489.
12. Potisek NM, McNeal-Trice K, Barone MA. The Whole "PROOF": Incorporating Evidence-Based Medicine Into Clinical Teaching. *Pediatrics*. 2017;140(1):e20171073. doi:10.1542/peds.2017-1073.

The Didactic Makeover: Keep it Short, Active, Relevant

Molly Rideout, MD,[a] Melissa Held, MD,[b] Alison Volpe Holmes, MD, MPH[c]

The test of a good teacher is not how many questions he can ask his pupils that they will answer readily, but how many questions he inspires them to ask him which he finds it hard to answer.[1]

Alice Wellington Rollins

Medical student education is rapidly evolving. Because students have immediate access to instant information online via high quality textbooks, research articles, lectures, and tutorials, the effectiveness of traditional lectures has come into question.[2–5] This presents an opportunity for pediatricians to develop new ways to deliver content to students. Teaching physicians in many institutions are developing interactive forms of learning, with some using entirely problem-based learning formats and others adapting traditional lectures into team-based learning or case-based presentations.[6,7] Stanford University has been a leader in this field for years and, in partnership with Khan Academy, has developed a program called Stanford Medicine Interactive Learning Initiatives, where medical school faculty can access specialized support to re-design courses and integrate interactive learning.[8] These large-scale initiatives are transforming the way students learn and how faculty members teach.

We continue the Council on Medical Student Education in Pediatrics series about great clinical teachers providing tools to keep educational sessions short, active, and relevant to engage students when refreshing or designing learning sessions .

KEEP IT SHORT

Retention of material varies with the length of the lesson. During learning sessions, students remember best what comes first, followed by what comes last, and retain the content presented in the middle the least.[9] Retention also varies with teaching method, with lectures producing the least amount of retention and teaching to others producing the greatest.[9]

Small Group Learning

Small group learning has been shown to increase students' ability to apply concepts versus learn about concepts.[10] As an alternative to a traditional 1-hour lecture, teachers can use the lecture's learning objectives and reformat them into topics for small group discussion. After a brief 10-minute introduction to a topic, students form small groups and discuss questions or clinical cases that have been created ahead of time. After students spend a set amount of time working through questions or cases, the facilitator elicits responses from the groups about ideas that surfaced during the discussions. Groups present their proposed answers and points of agreement or disagreement to learn together.

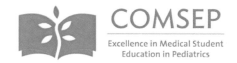

COMSEP
Excellence in Medical Student
Education in Pediatrics

[a]Department of Pediatrics, University of Vermont College of Medicine, Burlington, Vermont; [b]Department of Pediatrics, University of Connecticut School of Medicine, Farmington, Connecticut; and [c]Department of Pediatrics, Geisel School of Medicine at Dartmouth, Hanover, New Hampshire

Dr Rideout conceptualized the paper and drafted and revised the initial manuscript; Dr Held conceptualized the paper and reviewed and revised the manuscript; Dr Volpe Holmes conceptualized the paper and reviewed and revised the manuscript; and all authors approved the final manuscript as submitted.

DOI: 10.1542/peds.2016-0751

Accepted for publication Mar 15, 2016

Address correspondence to Molly Rideout, MD, Department of Pediatrics, University of Vermont Medical Center, MCHV Campus 265 SM5; 111 Colchester Ave, Burlington, VT 05401. E-mail: molly.rideout@uvmhealth.org

PEDIATRICS (ISSN Numbers: Print, 0031-4005; Online, 1098-4275).

FINANCIAL DISCLOSURE: The authors have indicated they have no financial relationships relevant to this article to disclose.

FUNDING: No external funding.

POTENTIAL CONFLICT OF INTEREST: The authors have indicated they have no potential conflicts of interest to disclose.

To cite: Rideout M, Held M, Holmes AV. The Didactic Makeover: Keep it Short, Active, Relevant. *Pediatrics.* 2016; 138(1):e20160751

Modified Team-based Learning

In traditional team-based learning, students read material ahead of time.[10] What happens if the students are not prepared? A modified team-based learning approach can be used. Students spend 10 minutes at the first part of a session reading over material individually before dividing into small groups. Original lecture slides can be used as is or adapted for students to review during the self-learning time. After reviewing information, students answer a series of multiple choice questions individually. Subsequently, they join into small groups to review and debate answers. During small group discussions, it is helpful for the teacher to allow the learning to happen without taking center stage, but acting as a "guide on the side".[3] As students process information and teach each other, even (and especially) working through mistakes, true learning occurs.[11] After working through questions, groups commit to answers (on paper, scratch cards, or audience response systems if available) and share with the larger group. If time permits, groups can debate 1 or 2 clinical application questions related to the topic.

By keeping it short, with didactic learning limited to 10 minutes at a time, students are more likely to stay focused and learn by applying the material to clinical cases.

KEEP IT ACTIVE

Students have a vast array of learning styles.[12,13] This can be beneficial for everyone; multiple people looking at the same problem in different ways may shed a clearer light on the entire picture and allow for better consolidation of learning.

Teachers need to be inclusive of different learning styles when designing educational sessions. Some key learning characteristics include active versus reflective and visual versus verbal.[12] A typical active learner might say, "let's try it out and see how it works," whereas a reflective learner might say, "let's think it through first." Visual learners learn best by seeing pictures, diagrams, or demonstrations, whereas verbal learners learn best by words, whether written or spoken. Most traditional lectures are geared toward reflective and verbal learners, but many learners are active and visual, which means it is challenging for them to stay engaged in traditional lectures.

Incorporating active learning into traditional presentations to include visual and active learners is relatively easy. Hands-on experiences, such as a field trip to the laboratory to look at slides or cultures, a visit from the respiratory therapist to demonstrate oxygen delivery systems, or taste testing medications or infant formulas, can keep students engaged.

Technology used in real-time is another way to keep learning active.[14] Students can pull up online videos of physical findings, such as stridor or paroxysmal cough, during presentations to their peers. Choosing a student to "find an answer" to another student's question during the session and teach the rest of the group is also engaging; this approach connects the group to

TABLE 1 Tools for Interactive Teaching

Active Learning Strategies	Teaching Modalities
Keep it short	Small groups
	10-min didactic
	Reformat learning objectives
	Prepare questions/cases
	Small group discussions
	Present back to larger group
	Modified team-based learning sessions
	Prepare fact sheet
	Prepare questions
	10-min self-learning
	Answer questions individually
	Small groups to discuss/debate questions
	Present back to larger group
Keep it active	Hands-on learning/field trips
	Laboratory: slides, cultures
	Respiratory therapist
	Medication/formula taste test
	Real-time technology
	Online videos (seizures, stridor)
	Online photos of physical findings
	Look up answers online in real-time
	Developing clinical questions
	Create (or have students create) clinical questions
	Find primary sources to answer clinical questions
	Present journal articles to group
Keep it relevant	Real patient/parent
	Brief introduction, guest shares story
	Leave time for questions and debriefing
	Be mindful of time constraints
	Simulation
	Work through cases in teams
	High fidelity: vital signs and exam findings change
	Low fidelity: verbal report or role play changes
	Case-based format
	Reorganize traditional lectures
	Clinical scenario for each section
	Factual material after each case
	Include photos/videos

the material and reflects the teacher's openness to questioning.

Students can investigate specific clinical questions during learning sessions by searching for journal articles individually or in small groups. Using explicit time limits, students can briefly present answers from primary sources without the expectation of a finished product. In this manner, they are exposed to the reality of having to quickly find studies to support a clinical decision.

KEEP IT RELEVANT

When clinical relevance is apparent, retention of material is likely to be higher.[2,4] Teachers can ensure relevance by including live patients, using simulation, or developing case-based scenarios.

Sometimes, a real patient or parent is available to visit during the session. After a brief introduction, the patient or parent can provide a short report of his or her medical experience either in the hospital, the clinic, or at home, leaving time for students to ask questions as well as to debrief following the visit. Orienting the family ahead of time about the learning goals of the session and any time constraints is essential.

Simulation is also an effective method to keep learning relevant.[15] Using high-fidelity simulators, students can work in teams developing clinical management skills in a realistic setting where clinical response to therapy change is based on team management decisions. If access to high-fidelity simulators is limited, teachers can use low-technology alternatives, such as dolls, with verbal report on changing symptoms and physical exam findings for diagnoses, such as croup or dehydration.

Another effective method to keep sessions patient-focused is

case-based learning.[16] Traditional presentations can be adapted fairly easily into a case-based format. By dividing content into a few areas, a clinical scenario or clinical question can be developed for each area, with factual material to follow. Time for discussion between cases to allow for questioning is helpful. If photos or videos are included in the presentation, the material will engage visual learners.

Teachers in different settings can use multiple strategies, adapting them as needed for use in outpatient clinics, inpatient wards, emergency departments, and subspecialty clinics. Creating a culture of shared learning, where learners feel free to solve problems and learn from "wrong" answers is 1 step toward effective learning.

Keeping learners engaged in this era of quick access to information and alternative educational modalities is challenging, but critical.[17] Teachers may find that "keeping it short, active, and relevant" is a useful mantra when designing educational sessions (Table 1).

REFERENCES

1. Winship AR. What they say. *Journal of Education*. 1898;47(22):339

2. Prober CG, Heath C. Lecture halls without lectures--a proposal for medical education. *N Engl J Med*. 2012;366(18):1657–1659

3. King A. From sage on the stage to guide on the side. *Coll Teach*. 1993;41(1)30–35

4. Mazur E. Education. Farewell, lecture? *Science*. 2009;323(5910):50–51

5. Berrett D. How 'flipping' the classroom can improve the traditional lecture. *The Chronicle of Higher Education*. February 19, 2012. Available at: http://chronicle.com/article/How-Flipping-the-Classroom/130857. Accessed October 12, 2015

6. Koles PG, Stolfi A, Borges NJ, Nelson S, Parmelee DX. The impact of team-based learning on medical students' academic performance. *Acad Med*. 2010;85(11):1739–1745

7. Koh GC, Khoo HE, Wong ML, Koh D. The effects of problem-based learning during medical school on physician competency: a systematic review. *CMAJ*. 2008;178(1):34–41

8. Stanford University. Stanford Medicine Interactive Learning Initiatives. Available at: smili.stanford.edu. Accessed October, 12, 2015

9. Sousa D. *How the Brain Learns*. 4th ed. Thousand Oaks, CA: Corwin; 2011

10. Michaelson LK, Parmelee DX, McMahon KK, et al. *Team Based Learning for Health Professions Education: A Guide to Using Small Groups for Improving Learning*. Sterling, VA: Stylus; 2008

11. Robinson K. Do schools kill creativity? Available at: www.ted.com/talks/ken_robinson_says_schools_kill_creativity?language=en. Accessed October 12, 2015

12. Felder RM, Silverman L. Learning and teaching styles in engineering education. *Engr Educ*. 1988;78(7):674–681

13. Kolb DA. *Experiential Learning: Experience as the Source of Learning and Development*. 2nd ed. New York: Pearson; 2015

14. Hines PJ, Jasny BR, Mervis J. Adding a T to the three R's. Education & technology. Introduction. *Science*. 2009;323(5910):53

15. Steadman RH, Coates WC, Huang YM, et al. Simulation-based training is superior to problem-based learning for the acquisition of critical assessment and management skills. *Crit Care Med*. 2006;34(1):151–157

16. Thistlethwaite JE, Davies D, Ekeocha S, et al. The effectiveness of case-based learning in health professional education. A BEME systematic review: BEME Guide No. 23. *Med Teach*. 2012;34(6):e421–e444

17. Musallam R. 3 rules to spark learning. Available at: www.ted.com/talks/ramsey_musallam_3_rules_to_spark_learning. Accessed October 12, 2015

Questioning as a Teaching Tool

Michele Long, MD[a], Rebecca Blankenburg, MD, MPH[b], Lavjay Butani, MD, MACM[c]

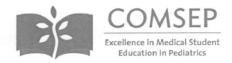

[a]Department of Pediatrics, University of California, San Francisco, San Francisco, California; [b]Department of Pediatrics, Stanford University School of Medicine, Stanford, California; and [c]Department of Pediatrics, University of California Davis Medical Center, Sacramento, California

Drs Long, Blankenburg, and Butani conceptualized the article and wrote the first draft of the article. All authors contributed to the literature search, reviewed and revised the manuscript, and approved the final manuscript as submitted.

www.pediatrics.org/cgi/doi/10.1542/peds.2014-3285

DOI: 10.1542/peds.2014-3285

Accepted for publication Oct 15, 2014

Address correspondence to Michele Long, MD, Department of Pediatrics, University of California, San Francisco, 513 Parnassus Ave, San Francisco, CA 94143. E-mail: michele.long@ucsf.edu

PEDIATRICS (ISSN Numbers: Print, 0031-4005; Online, 1098-4275).

FINANCIAL DISCLOSURE: The authors have indicated they have no financial relationships relevant to this article to disclose.

FUNDING: No external funding.

POTENTIAL CONFLICT OF INTEREST: The authors have indicated they have no potential conflicts of interest to disclose.

Questions are a central part of the practice, and teaching, of medicine. Through questioning, we diagnose patients, reflect upon our own practice, assess learners, and teach. This article provides an approach to questioning for the purposes of student assessment and teaching by considering the Dreyfus and Bloom frameworks. The authors offer practical ways to use questions to diagnose students' understanding, to teach, and to model life-long learning.

Susan Bannister, Editor-in-Chief, Council on Medical Student Education in Pediatrics Monthly Feature

This article is part of the Council on Medical Student Education in Pediatrics series on strategies and techniques used by great clinical teachers. Herein we explore how educators can best use questioning strategies to promote learning in the clinical setting. Teachers commonly ask questions to assess learners' knowledge.[1,2] When used strategically, questioning can engage learners by stimulating active participation in the learning process, guide them toward the understanding of deeper concepts, promote peer–peer collaboration, and build their confidence.[1] Moreover, through questioning, clinicians can stimulate critical thinking while actively modeling the process of inquiry and life-long learning.[1]

Questioning is a challenging teaching tool and even experienced, well-meaning educators occasionally make mistakes. Teachers often rely heavily on recall-based questions that fail to stimulate deeper thinking and can cause learners to disengage.[3,4] Questions that are mismatched to learner level can be equally problematic; asking novice learners unrealistically challenging questions can lead them to lose self-confidence and interest and asking advanced learners fact-based questions can demotivate them. Finally, questions posed in a seemingly confrontational manner (which can cause anxiety in learners and may be perceived as "pimping") can adversely affect the learning climate.[1,5] We provide a framework for matching questions to a learner's ability and provide suggestions for formulating questions to both challenge learners and maintain a supportive learning environment.

CONSTRUCTING QUESTIONS BASED ON LEARNER ABILITY

Different learners and teaching situations require different types of questions. One approach to effective questioning takes into consideration the developmental stage of the learner and the learning objectives best suited for the stage.

The educator first classifies the developmental stage of the learner based on his or her competence, confidence, and motivation by using the Dreyfus model of skills acquisition.[6] The 4 Dreyfus stages most relevant to clinical educators are novice (learners function by using a limited rule-based knowledge system without a clinical context), advanced beginner (learners have an expanded repertoire of clinical rules and may just be getting exposed to a clinical environment), competent (learners use rules of thumb and are in the process of getting invested in the actual care of their patients), and proficient (learners show increasing initiative in patient care and use intuitive clinical reasoning based on their previously gained clinical experience).[6] Generally, most students will be in the novice to advanced beginner stage, whereas most residents will be in the advanced beginner to competent stage. Some residents and many fellows may be in the proficient phase, but few are likely to be at the higher stages of expert or master and these stages are not addressed in this article.[6] These generalizations can break down for some trainees (such as a particularly experienced medical student) and in some situations (such as a senior resident encountering a patient with a specific or rare disease for the first time). Therefore, getting to know your learner by asking about their background and experiences and probing their knowledge base is very important.[7]

The next step is to think about the type of question to ask, by matching the assessed developmental level of the learner to the learning objectives for that stage of learner.[1,2,8] One framework for formulating specific questions matched to each of the learner levels uses Bloom's taxonomy.[1,2,6,8] Bloom's taxonomy is a hierarchy widely used by educators that places thinking skills at 6 levels: knowledge (lowest level), comprehension, application, analysis, synthesis, and evaluation (highest level).[2,8] The most relevant to clinical questioning of students and residents are the levels from knowledge to analysis. Due to limited clinical experience, novice learners benefit most from simple questions focused on factual knowledge.[1] These questions are often phrased in a direct manner and have a single best answer. Advanced beginner learners are working on linking facts they may have learned in isolation, so questions should prompt them to connect information and demonstrate understanding of concepts and comprehension. Competent and proficient learners are applying information to common clinical situations, so questions can be more complex and prompt them to apply theoretical knowledge to a specific clinical situation in the decision-making process. Learners can be asked to analyze a situation or to compare and contrast 2 or more options for managing a patient's medical issues. Questions may also pose alternatives to what the learner proposed, followed by an exploration of their thought process. Specific examples of questions using the Bloom framework matched to developmental stage (Dreyfus) are listed in Table 1.

Although fact-based questions are good for building confidence and assessing knowledge, especially for novice learners, clinical teachers should avoid the common pitfall of relying on "low level" questions promoting rote memorization without true understanding of concepts.[1,3,4] Even with novice learners, one can use a step-up approach and ask increasingly complex follow-up questions to simultaneously engage and challenge learners and create "constructive friction,"[9] provided questioning does not become too challenging or intimidating.[2] For more advanced learners, questioning can start at a higher level and be open-ended, with a step-down to simpler questions if learners struggle finding answers.[2] In groups or with multiple levels of learners, such as on ward rounds, it is often easiest to begin the questioning process directed toward the primary learner taking care of the patient. However, remember to keep the group engaged by asking questions of all or several of the team members, matched to their developmental level.[2]

QUESTIONING WHILE MAINTAINING A POSITIVE LEARNING ENVIRONMENT

Although questioning inherently puts the learner "on-the-spot," it is possible to minimize discomfort while promoting a positive learning environment. First, set the expectation with learners that you will be asking questions. Explain that your goal is to explore their

TABLE 1 Asking Questions Based on Learner Developmental Level

Developmental Stage of Learner (Dreyfus)	Objectives for Questions to Focus on (Bloom)	Goal of Questioning	Stems to Consider Using	Sample Question(s): Based on a Patient With a Possible Urinary Tract Infection
Novice	Knowledge	Build knowledge	List Define Name	List the 3 ways a specimen can be obtained for urine culture. What are the diagnostic criteria for a urinary tract infection?
Advanced beginner	Comprehension	Promote understanding of concepts	Explain Describe	Explain why a urine culture is indicated in a febrile infant.
Competent	Application	Stimulate application of knowledge to a clinical context	Interpret	Here is our patient's urinalysis … what do you think this tells us and why (or interpret these results)?
Proficient	Analysis	Break down complex concepts into their component parts	Compare and Contrast	Compare and contrast the need for a urine culture in a febrile male infant and a febrile female teenager, both without localizing signs and symptoms.

understanding and build upon what they already know.[1,2]

Great clinical teachers pay particular attention to how questions are asked. They avoid asking questions in a rapid-fire sequence, and instead ask questions one at a time. Allowing learners between 3 and 5 seconds to respond with an answer has been shown to increase both the likelihood of getting a response and also the length of the response.[2,10] Importantly, avoid interrupting learners while they are formulating a response and wait after receiving a response before asking a follow-up question.[1]

To further promote a positive learning environment, teachers can ask open-ended questions that increase the chance of their learner being able to find an acceptable answer, on which they can then elaborate ("Can you explain to the team your thought process?").[11] The teacher can also restate the learner's answer to confirm respect for his or her thoughts ("You've brought up a good point …"). In a group setting, directing questions to other learners on the team can simultaneously reduce the pressure on the learner who is presenting information and engage others in learning. Getting a commitment on the same question from all learners before revealing the answer is another way to involve the entire team in the learning process. Finally, resist the temptation to provide answers to all of the learners' questions; challenge learners to research the question and report back.

If the learner's response to a question seems noncommittal or is incorrect, guide them while maintaining

confidence in their abilities, especially in front of patients. As alluded to earlier, this is another time when open-ended brief clarifying questions can be asked instead of answering the question or turning to others ("Can you tell us more about that?").[1,11] Similarly, when a learner is initially incorrect, guiding them to the correct answer by using a gentle approach is a way to challenge learners without humiliating them ("That's an interesting thought. If that was the diagnosis, how would you explain the absence of…?").[12]

Lastly, if the opportunity arises, think about asking the learners themselves to generate and pose questions to the team, to further engage them. These can then be researched individually or as a group and discussed the next time the team comes together.

SUMMARY

The Dreyfus and Bloom frameworks can help the great clinical teacher craft questions that are learner-centric and appropriately challenging. Employing strategies to ask the right questions in the right way can further add to the effectiveness of using questions as a valuable teaching, learning, and assessment tool.

ACKNOWLEDGMENTS

The authors thank Drs Robert Dudas, Christopher Maloney, and Susan Bannister for their thoughtful review and editing of the article.

REFERENCES

1. Tofade T, Elsner J, Haines ST. Best practice strategies for effective use of questions as a teaching tool. *Am J Pharm Educ*. 2013;77(7):155

2. Sachdeva AK. Use of effective questioning to enhance the cognitive abilities of students. *J Cancer Educ*. 1996;11(1):17–24

3. Phillips N, Duke M. The questioning skills of clinical teachers and preceptors: a comparative study. *J Adv Nurs*. 2001;33(4):523–529

4. Sellappah S, Hussey T, Blackmore AM, McMurray A. The use of questioning strategies by clinical teachers. *J Adv Nurs*. 1998;28(1):142–148

5. Brancati FL. The art of pimping. *JAMA*. 1989;262(1):89–90

6. Carraccio CL, Benson BJ, Nixon LJ, Derstine PL. From the educational bench to the clinical bedside: translating the Dreyfus developmental model to the learning of clinical skills. *Acad Med*. 2008;83(8):761–767

7. Raszka WV Jr, Maloney CG, Hanson JL. Getting off to a good start: discussing goals and expectations with medical students. *Pediatrics*. 2010;126(2):193–195

8. Bloom BS. *Taxonomy of Educational Objectives: The Classification of Educational Goals: Handbook I: Cognitive Domain*. New York, NY: David McKay Company, Inc; 1956

9. ten Cate O, Snell L, Mann K, Vermunt J. Orienting teaching toward the learning process. *Acad Med*. 2004;79(3):219–228

10. Schneider JR, Sherman HB, Prystowsky JB, Schindler N, Darosa DA. Questioning skills: the effect of wait time on accuracy of medical student responses to oral and written questions. *Acad Med*. 2004;79(suppl 10):S28–S31

11. Spencer J. Learning and teaching in the clinical environment. *BMJ*. 2003;326(7389):591–594

12. Ramani S. Twelve tips to improve bedside teaching. *Med Teach*. 2003;25(2):112–115

Transform Role Modeling Into SUPERmodeling

Nicholas M. Potisek, MD,[a] Barrett Fromme, MD, MHPE,[b] Michael S. Ryan, MD[c]

Role modeling is the process by which a learner observes a clinical teacher to develop and refine his or her practice. Compared to other learning methods, role modeling is inherently student driven and may occur with or without the clinical teacher's awareness.[1,2] Perhaps this is why learners often experience poor role modeling behaviors,[2] and clinician teachers struggle to identify role modeling opportunities.[3] Although role modeling is traditionally considered a passive or implicit learning method, newer evidence suggests clinical teachers can transform the role modeling process into a more explicit teaching method to enhance the development of their leaners.[2,4]

IMPORTANCE

Clinical teachers serve a critical role in shaping attitudes and behaviors of future generations of physicians. Role modeling can be effectively used to teach challenging clinical skills such as verbal and nonverbal communication, humanism, professionalism, and teamwork.[1] Role modeling may also be the most effective and efficient learning method in busy clinical environments or when a patient care task is beyond the learner's current clinical abilities.[5] A learner's observations of the clinician teacher's behaviors may influence his or her professional development and career

decisions.[5,6] Unfortunately, not all experiences are positive. Learners commonly witness unprofessional behavior and report difficulty identifying positive role models.[7] Furthermore, learners may perceive observation experiences as "shadowing" and may subscribe less value to these opportunities than seeing patients independently. A clinical teacher's ability to role model effectively and explicitly can significantly enhance the learner experience and his or her development into a clinician.

TOOLS AND TIPS

In this article from the Council on Medical Students in Pediatrics series on great clinical teachers, we offer specific strategies for transforming role modeling into SUPERmodeling. The SUPER mnemonic (increasing self-awareness, helping the unconscious become conscious, plan debriefing, and encourage reflection) provides clinical teachers with a toolbox to enhance role modeling strategies. These strategies are summarized in Fig 1. To demonstrate each, we will provide illustrative examples through the following clinical teacher-learner dyad: Dr Paul is a busy community-based pediatrician. She is an excellent clinician continuously seeking ways to improve her teaching. Dr Paul decides to focus on developing her role modeling skills in various clinical encounters with

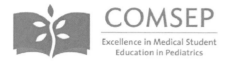

[a]Department of Pediatrics, Wake Forest School of Medicine, Winston-Salem, North Carolina; [b]Department of Pediatrics, Pritzker School of Medicine, University of Chicago, Chicago, Illinois; and [c]Department of Pediatrics, School of Medicine, Virginia Commonwealth University, Richmond, Virginia

Drs Potisek, Fromme, and Ryan conceptualized and designed the manuscript, drafted the initial manuscript, and reviewed and revised the manuscript; and all authors approved the final manuscript as submitted and agree to be accountable for all aspects of the work.

DOI: https://doi.org/10.1542/peds.2019-2624

Accepted for publication Aug 13, 2019

Address correspondence to Nicholas M. Potisek, MD, Department of Pediatrics, Wake Forest School of Medicine, Medical Center Blvd, Winston-Salem, NC 27157. E-mail: npotisek@wakehealth.edu

PEDIATRICS (ISSN Numbers: Print, 0031-4005; Online, 1098-4275).

FINANCIAL DISCLOSURE: The authors have indicated they have no financial relationships relevant to this article to disclose.

FUNDING: No external funding.

POTENTIAL CONFLICT OF INTEREST: The authors have indicated they have no potential conflicts of interest to disclose. The authors have no potential conflicts of interest to disclose.

To cite: Potisek NM, Fromme B, Ryan MS. Transform Role Modeling Into SUPERmodeling. *Pediatrics.* 2019;144(5): e20192624

a third-year medical student by the name of Taylor who is coming to her office for the next month.

Self-awareness

Extraordinary role modeling begins by increasing the clinical teacher's self-awareness of their influence on learners.[1,2,8] Clinician teachers continuously model behaviors and must therefore recognize their influence on learner behaviors in all circumstances. An increased self-awareness can prompt clinical teachers to anticipate and identify clinical scenarios to incorporate role modeling into practice and to identify specific objectives from each patient encounter.[8] Discussing this responsibility with learners can help hold clinical teachers accountable for their actions and heighten their own awareness of their impact on learners.

Illustrative Example:

Previous learners have praised Dr Paul's ability to navigate challenging patient conversations. As a result, she is more mindful of clinical scenarios a learner may view as challenging. She identifies vaccine-hesitant families, concerns for child abuse, and situations of medical uncertainty as potential role modeling opportunities. On the first day of the rotation, Dr Paul relays to Taylor there will be opportunities to see patients directly and observe Dr Paul's bedside manner. She describes the benefits of both experiences.

Unconscious Becomes Conscious

The impact of learning through role modeling is dependent on the learner's awareness, engagement, and accurate assessment of the observed behavior.[2,9,10] On occasion, a learner may unconsciously incorporate an observed behavior without fully understanding the clinical teacher's intent.[2,10] This may result in the learner modifying his or her practice in a way that is detrimental. Therefore, addressing unconscious

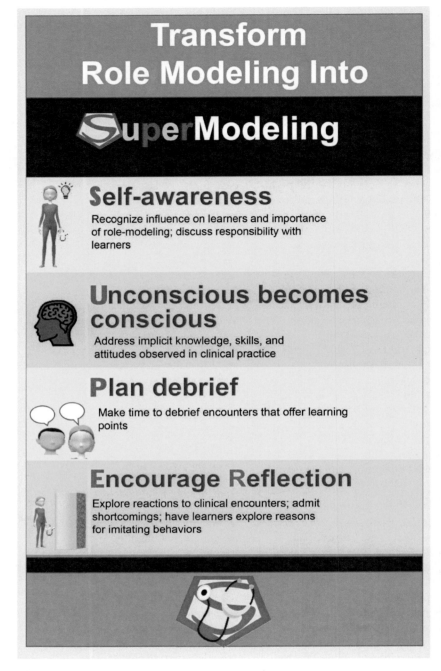

FIGURE 1
Four strategies to transform role modeling into SUPERmodeling.

elements of learning in role modeling is essential to ensure learners thoughtfully include or exclude observed behaviors into their own practice. Clinical teachers can do this by preparing the learner in advance for what they will observe and how

the clinician plans to navigate the situation.

Illustrative Example

The mother of a 12-month-old patient well known to Dr Paul is hesitant about vaccination. The patient is scheduled for a routine follow-up with Dr Paul. Dr Paul takes a moment to recall how challenging such encounters can be for a new clinician and identifies this interaction as a good opportunity for Taylor to observe. After sharing the background perspective, Dr Paul presents her planned approach to navigate today's discussion and her rationale behind this approach. She asks Taylor to actively observe and create his own perspective on how the encounter goes.

Plan Debriefing

Because role modeling is often viewed as a passive process, an intentional debrief is not generally considered a core component of this teaching method.[1] This is grounded in the assumption that learners will accurately recognize the rationale behind a clinical teacher's behavior. However, this approach is susceptible to misinterpretation, particularly during difficult encounters. In situations such as these, role modeling may be enhanced by incorporating a more explicit and planned debrief. The purpose of a planned debrief is for the clinical teacher to discuss why they used a certain behavior or particular language and to address the learner's reaction.[2] Clinical teachers may highlight the motivation for a behavior by including previous experiences and why they favor the observed approach.

Illustrative Example

Dr Paul debriefs with Taylor after their previous patient encounter. She asks Taylor to describe observations from the interaction between Dr Paul and the mother. Taylor articulates observations regarding verbal and nonverbal communication and mentions being surprised Dr Paul was not more assertive regarding the need to vaccinate the infant. Dr Paul shares her perspective on the value of building a therapeutic relationship with families in hopes that, over time,

she would be able to change the mother's perspective on vaccines.

Encourage Reflection

Reflection on part of both the clinical teacher and learner helps reveal the implicit benefits of role modeling.[9] Before patient encounters, clinical teachers can encourage learners to not just adapt or abstain from clinical behaviors they witness but to explore their own reactions and reasons for imitating certain clinical behaviors. The clinician can take the lead on demonstrating reflection by readily admitting shortcomings and/or clinical uncertainty to reinforce a learning environment conducive to self-reflection. Engaging learners in such conversations can promote the need for self-reflection throughout a career.

Illustrative Example

Two days ago, a patient Dr Paul had referred for subspecialty evaluation returned to her clinic. Dr Paul was disappointed in the evaluation the subspecialist provided and voiced her displeasure to Taylor. Today, Dr Paul intentionally sat down with Taylor to acknowledge that she had been impatient the previous afternoon and had wanted to advocate for her patient, not disrespect the subspecialist. She expressed regret to the learner in the way she talked about the subspecialist. She asked how Taylor might have done things differently in his own practice in the future.

CONCLUSIONS

Role modeling is a powerful teaching strategy. Clinician teachers can make role modeling SUPERmodeling through incorporating the various teaching components of increasing self-awareness, making the unconscious more conscious, plan debriefing, and encourage reflection. Ideally, all 4 role modeling teaching strategies can be used in a given clinical encounter; however, even in

isolation, the use of any of these strategies can enhance a clinical teacher's ability to role model.

ABBREVIATION

SUPER: increasing self-awareness, helping the unconscious become conscious, plan debriefing, and encourage reflection

---

REFERENCES

1. Weissmann PF, Branch WT, Gracey CF, Haidet P, Frankel RM. Role modeling humanistic behavior: learning bedside manner from the experts. *Acad Med.* 2006;81(7):661–667

2. Cruess SR, Cruess RL, Steinert Y. Role modelling–making the most of a powerful teaching strategy. *BMJ.* 2008;336(7646):718–721

3. Côté L, Leclère H. How clinical teachers perceive the doctor-patient relationship and themselves as role models. *Acad Med.* 2000;75(11):1117–1124

4. Kenny NP, Mann KV, MacLeod H. Role modeling in physicians' professional formation: reconsidering an essential but untapped educational strategy. *Acad Med.* 2003;78(12):1203–1210

5. Yoon JD, Ham SA, Reddy ST, Curlin FA. Role models' influence on specialty choice for residency training: a national longitudinal study. *J Grad Med Educ.* 2018;10(2):149–154

6. Wright S, Wong A, Newill C. The impact of role models on medical students. *J Gen Intern Med.* 1997;12(1):53–56

7. Wright S. Examining what residents look for in their role models. *Acad Med.* 1996;71(3):290–292

8. Wright SM, Carrese JA. Excellence in role modelling: insight and perspectives from the pros. *CMAJ.* 2002;167(6):638–643

9. Benbassat J. Role modeling in medical education: the importance of a reflective imitation. *Acad Med.* 2014;89(4):550–554

10. Epstein RM, Cole DR, Gawinski BA, Piotrowski-Lee S, Ruddy NB. How students learn from community-based preceptors. *Arch Fam Med.* 1998;7(2):149–154

Failure Is an Option: Using Errors as Teaching Opportunities

Jimmy B. Beck, MD, MEd, Caitlin McGrath, MD, Kristina Toncray, MD, Sahar N. Rooholamini, MD, MPH

Success consists of going from failure to failure without loss of enthusiasm.

Winston Churchill

In this article, we continue the Council on Medical Student Education in Pediatrics series describing the characteristics and skills of effective clinical teachers by providing a practical framework for using errors as opportunities to promote the professional growth of students. For our purposes, a medical error is "the failure of a planned action to be completed as intended or the use of a wrong plan to achieve an aim."[1]

Because medical students are closely supervised during their clinical rotations, it is unlikely that a student error would lead to major patient harm. However, many students will experience an error during medical school[2] and may be reluctant to report their own errors for fear of negatively impacting their evaluations.[3] The hidden curriculum, which refers to the implicit culture of rules and norms present in the clinical learning environment, may also discourage a student from speaking up.[4] Furthermore, students who have a negative experience after an error occurs are less likely to take responsibility for future errors, [5] whereas students who witness their attending physicians take ownership of errors are more likely to emulate that behavior.[6]

Rather than minimizing errors, great clinical teachers acknowledge errors as opportunities to teach students to reflect and take helpful action.[4] Despite the potential benefits of using errors as teaching opportunities, barriers such as time constraints, the desire to avoid uncomfortable future relationships with students, and a lack of training about how to make disclosures may make physicians hesitant to discuss errors with students.[7]

The following 3-part framework is helpful for transforming medical errors into valuable learning opportunities: (1) orient students to errors as learning opportunities, (2) model appropriate ways to view and handle errors, and (3) debrief errors with students. We share a fictional case to illustrate this framework:

You are supervising Elaine, a third-year medical student on her pediatric clerkship, in a busy outpatient clinic. She feels a sense of satisfaction with her Spanish-speaking skills after interviewing and examining a non-English–speaking patient with vomiting and makes a diagnosis of acute gastroenteritis. When you interview the patient using a certified interpreter, you note that key elements are missing from the history, and on your examination, the patient has examination findings classic for appendicitis.

ORIENT

Effective learning requires clear expectations within an emotionally supportive environment.[8] Establishing a framework for

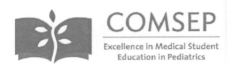

Department of Pediatrics, University of Washington, Seattle, Washington

Dr Beck and Dr Rooholamini conceptualized the ideas presented and drafted the initial manuscript; Drs McGrath and Toncray conceptualized the ideas presented; and all authors reviewed and revised the manuscript and approved the final manuscript as submitted.

DOI: https://doi.org/10.1542/peds.2017-4222

Accepted for publication Dec 19, 2017

Address correspondence to Jimmy B. Beck, MD, MEd, Seattle Children's Hospital, 4800 Sandpoint Way NE, M/S FA.2.115, PO Box 5371, Seattle, WA 98105. E-mail: jimmy.beck@seattlechildrens.org

PEDIATRICS (ISSN Numbers: Print, 0031-4005; Online, 1098-4275).

FINANCIAL DISCLOSURE: The authors have indicated they have no financial relationships relevant to this article to disclose.

FUNDING: No external funding.

POTENTIAL CONFLICT OF INTEREST: The authors have indicated they have no potential conflicts of interest to disclose.

To cite: Beck JB, McGrath C, Toncray K, et al. Failure Is an Option: Using Errors as Teaching Opportunities. *Pediatrics.* 2018;141(3):e20174222

approaching errors intentionally and honestly establishes the teacher as a "safe" person with whom to discuss errors. Before the rotation begins, teachers can inform students about their own approach to discussing errors. When meeting students, teachers can reiterate their philosophy toward errors and ask students about their experiences with the disclosure of errors. Understanding a student's experience with errors establishes a baseline for future growth.

In Elaine's case, before the start of her rotation, you sent her an introductory email stating, among other things, "In my clinical work, I like to take a proactive approach when any error occurs. Errors are a normal part of clinical practice, with each error providing a valuable opportunity to improve."

MODEL

Many students have not observed a teacher modeling the disclosure and discussion of errors.[9]

Modeling a professional response to errors requires the willingness to be vulnerable. Modeling of vulnerability by the teacher through open discussion with the team, patients, and families after an error is associated with positive learner attitudes and behaviors, such as accepting responsibility for and disclosing errors.[10] When teachers discuss lessons and growth from their errors, students may gain a better understanding of how to approach their own errors.[4,11]

DEBRIEF ERRORS

The final component of using errors as teaching opportunities involves intentional debriefing after students witness or are involved in an error. The acronym I-HELP (introduction, homework, emotional support, learning) (Table 1) provides a structure for teachers to use to guide students through debriefing an error.

TABLE 1 Guidelines for Debriefing Errors With Medical Students: I-HELP Acronym

I-HELP Guidelines
1. Introduction
Set the expectation during orientation that errors are a part of medical practice and will be treated as valuable learning opportunities.
Model an appropriate response to your own mistakes.
2. Homework
Assess: Do you have rapport with this student? Are you the most appropriate person to debrief with the student?
Determine the appropriate timing on the basis of student preference (eg, immediate versus delayed timing). Would the student benefit from some time to self-reflect before debriefing?
Choose the appropriate setting. Private settings are usually most appropriate, although exceptions could be made, depending on factors such as the student's reaction to the error, the type of error, and the potential learning value.
"I think this is something that every team member has the potential to experience, would it be okay with you if we discussed this in a team setting so that we could all learn from it?"
3. Emotional support
Validate feelings and emotions.
"Thanks for meeting with me today. I know talking about errors can be hard. This discussion is not meant to be punitive. We are here to discuss what happened and how we can learn from it."
Avoid minimizing or dismissing the seriousness of the mistake; instead, help the student put it in perspective
"Unfortunately, this mistake occurred and resulted in patient harm; it's our responsibility to learn from it."
Be willing to share your own relevant stories of error.
"When I was a student, I had a similar experience and I felt . . . ."
4. Learning
Ask the student to articulate the main issue; what happened?
Celebrate successes.
"Before we talk about what didn't go well, can you think of what did go well?"
Focus on just 1 learning point, such as, "What did the student learn from this situation?"
"If a situation like this occurs again, what might we do differently?"
5. Plan for the future
Thank the student.
Discuss other available support resources.
"Do you have someone else to talk to about this for support?"
Offer to discuss the issue at any time.
"Please let me know if you would like to talk about this again."

Introduction

As above, before the occurrence of an error, teachers (1) set the expectation and then (2) model error discussion and disclosure as part of clinical practice and as valuable learning opportunities.

Homework

Clinical teachers prepare by considering the who, when, and where of error debriefing. In determining the most appropriate person to debrief with the student, a teacher considers whether they were directly involved with, or observed, the error. The teacher also reflects on whether they have a strong emotional response to the error. In some cases, another teacher or clerkship director may be a more appropriate person to debrief. Next, the teacher considers the appropriate timing, such as immediate or delayed timing. In general, feedback close in time to the event is preferable, although patient care may preclude an immediate discussion, and a student's emotional state plays a role in timing. Finally, choosing an appropriate setting is critical for building trust with the student.

During lunch, you ask Elaine to discuss the appendicitis case. You noticed that she did not seem surprised when you approached her and seemed open to further conversation.

Emotional Support

Given the significant emotional turmoil associated with committing an error,[11] it is critical to assess and validate the student's feelings. Avoid minimizing or dismissing the seriousness of the mistake. Instead, help the student gain perspective. Also, consider assessing for other support structures (ie, family, institutional support, others with similar experiences). Teachers can reduce the student's sense of isolation by sharing their own relevant stories of error and how they felt at the time.

Thanks for meeting with me today. I wanted to discuss our patient with appendicitis and the factors that may have led to initially missing the diagnosis. I know talking about errors can be hard. I remember missing a diagnosis when I was a student, and my attending correcting me but not really discussing it in the moment, which seemed like a lost opportunity to learn.

Learning

When sitting down to discuss, teachers use open-ended questions and ask the student to first articulate the event and then identify the main issue(s). This promotes guided self-reflection and allows the teacher to assess the student's state of mind. It can be helpful to ask students to articulate what they felt went well with the situation and reaffirm the successful aspects of their care. Lastly, teachers ask their students to discuss what they want to learn from the error, attempting to focus on 1 learning point.

When reflecting on today's patient, what do you think went well? How did this experience make you feel? What did you learn from this patient and your experience?

Plan for the Future

The teacher ends by thanking the student and offering to discuss the issue again at any time.

Elaine, thanks for being open to talking about this. Discussing and learning from

our errors can make people feel vulnerable, but it is part of how we grow as clinicians. My door is always open to you to talk more if you'd like.

Bridging or prompting statements such as the examples suggested in Table 1 can be used to promote trust and build support.

CONCLUSIONS

There are many missed opportunities to teach students how to respond to and learn from errors. Great clinical teachers can model proactive and intentional responses to errors, and by creating a supportive environment, they can guide students to process and learn from mistakes. Students who learn to discuss and grow from errors promote positive changes in their own professional development and, potentially, impact the health of their future patients.

ACKNOWLEDGMENTS

We thank Emily Ruedinger and Khiet Ngo for their help in conceptualizing this framework. We also thank Khiet Ngo for his helpful comments and thoughtful reviews of the article.

ABBREVIATION

I-HELP: introduction, homework, emotional support, learning

REFERENCES

1. Institute of Medicine (US) Committee on Quality of Health Care in America; Kohn LT, Corrigan JM, Donaldson MS, eds. *To Err Is Human: Building a Safer Health System*. Washington, DC: National Academy Press; 2000

2. Kiesewetter J, Kager M, Lux R, Zwissler B, Fischer MR, Dietz I. German undergraduate medical students' attitudes and needs regarding medical errors and patient safety–a national survey in Germany. *Med Teach*. 2014;36(6):505–510

3. Gold KB. *Medical Students' Exposure and Response to Error on the Ward*. New Haven, CT: Yale University; 2009

4. Fischer MA, Mazor KM, Baril J, Alper E, DeMarco D, Pugnaire M. Learning from mistakes. Factors that influence how students and residents learn from medical errors. *J Gen Intern Med*. 2006;21(5):419–423

5. Vohra PD, Johnson JK, Daugherty CK, Wen M, Barach P. Housestaff and medical student attitudes toward medical errors and adverse events. *Jt Comm J Qual Patient Saf*. 2007;33(8):493–501

6. Martinez W, Lo B. Medical students' experiences with medical errors: an analysis of medical student essays. *Med Educ*. 2008;42(7):733–741

7. Mazor KM, Fischer MA, Haley HL, Hatem D, Rogers HJ, Quirk ME. Factors influencing preceptors' responses to medical errors: a factorial survey. *Acad Med*. 2005;80(suppl 10):S88–S92

8. Bannister SL, Hanson JL, Maloney CG, Dudas RA. Practical framework for fostering a positive learning environment. *Pediatrics*. 2015;136(1):6–9

9. Bell SK, Moorman DW, Delbanco T. Improving the patient, family, and clinician experience after harmful events: the "when things go wrong" curriculum. *Acad Med*. 2010;85(6):1010–1017

10. Martinez W, Hickson GB, Miller BM, et al. Role-modeling and medical error disclosure: a national survey of trainees. *Acad Med*. 2014;89(3):482–489

11. Plews-Ogan M, May N, Owens J, Ardelt M, Shapiro J, Bell SK. Wisdom in medicine: what helps physicians after a medical error? *Acad Med*. 2016;91(2):233–241

Just Do It: Incorporating Bedside Teaching Into Every Patient Encounter

Susan L. Bannister, MD, Med, FRCPC,[a] Janice L. Hanson, PhD, EdS,[b] Christopher G. Maloney, MD, PhD,[c] Robert Arthur Dudas, MD[d]

He who studies medicine without books sails an uncharted sea, but he who studies medicine without patients does not go to sea at all.

William Osler

Students learn what it means to be a doctor at the bedside. Communication, professionalism, clinical reasoning, and the physical examination are best learned in the presence of patients. In this setting, students are able to make connections and apply what they learned in the classroom to the patient who is with them.

In this article, we continue the series by the Council on Medical Student Education in Pediatrics in which the skills and strategies used by great clinical teachers are described. In previous articles, we considered specific strategies to teach family-centered care,[1] clinical reasoning,[2] and humanism[3] at the bedside of patients. In this article, we provide practical tips to help busy clinicians incorporate bedside teaching into inpatient and outpatient care.

In our age of time pressures in clinical settings, multitasking, and short attention spans, clinical teachers face a challenging situation: how can they grab and maintain their learners' focus during patient encounters? The great news is that short clinical teaching at the bedside is likely to captivate students because they have become accustomed to communicating through texts and tweets. We reframe the challenge of "not having time to teach" to finding content for timely teaching; in just a few minutes, great clinical lessons can be taught from every bedside.

PREPARE YOURSELF AND YOUR TEAM

Experienced clinical teachers consult their patient list in advance and think about short teaching points based on the patients they will encounter in the clinic or during rounds. With these potential teaching points in mind, great clinical teachers focus their attention on creating a comfortable learning environment.[4] They may search for and print clinical guidelines or review articles for their students. Preparation, however, is primarily about getting in a positive frame of mind and walking into patient encounters with an open mind, ready to see (and seize) learning opportunities.

Clinical teachers prepare students for bedside teaching in several ways: they ensure introductions are made so that learners can identify others and their roles; they ask students if there are particular skills for which they would like to receive feedback; they remind their teams to simultaneously attend to the family's and patient's responses and that teaching sessions may vary in length or end abruptly, depending on what unfolds;

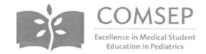

[a]University of Calgary, Calgary, Canada; [b]School of Medicine, University of Colorado, Aurora, Colorado; [c]University of Nebraska, Lincoln, Nebraska; and [d]School of Medicine, Johns Hopkins University, Baltimore, Maryland

DOI: https://doi.org/10.1542/peds.2018-1238

Accepted for publication Apr 20, 2018

Address correspondence to Robert Arthur Dudas, MD, Department of Pediatrics, Johns Hopkins All Children's Hospital, 601 5th St South, Suite 606, St Petersburg, FL 33701. E-mail: rdudas@jhmi.edu

PEDIATRICS (ISSN Numbers: Print, 0031-4005; Online, 1098-4275).

FINANCIAL DISCLOSURE: The authors have indicated they have no financial relationships relevant to this article to disclose.

FUNDING: No external funding.

POTENTIAL CONFLICT OF INTEREST: The authors have indicated they have no potential conflicts of interest to disclose.

To cite: Bannister SL, Hanson JL, Maloney CG, et al. Just Do It: Incorporating Bedside Teaching Into Every Patient Encounter. *Pediatrics.* 2018;142(1):e20181238

they outline guidelines for which information should not be discussed in front of the patient and family; they orient their learners to their teaching style; and they commit to not embarrassing their learners and tell them they will use a phrase such as "Let me show you another way to do that" if a student does something incorrectly.

COMPARE AND CONTRAST

As you see patients together, ask your learners to compare different diagnoses or the same diagnosis in different ages or types of patients. Consider the following questions that could be asked during an encounter with a patient in respiratory distress:

- How does this child's respiratory examination differ from the examination of our patient who has croup?

- Which clues from the physical examination make us suspect this infant has pertussis? What would make us think of bronchiolitis?

- What would you consider if this child had been coughing for only a few hours? For a few weeks?

- How would the respiratory examination be different if this child was an infant? An adolescent?

- How would this disease present if this infant had a congenital heart defect?

DON'T LIMIT YOUR TEACHING TO THE REASON(S) THE PATIENT IS IN THE HOSPITAL OR CLINIC

Great clinical teachers see teaching and learning opportunities everywhere. They are not restricted to discussing the disease of the patient before them.

Teach About Anticipatory Guidance

Use your clinical encounters to model and teach anticipatory guidance. If an infant is sleeping with a bottle in his or her bed, capitalize on the opportunity to discuss sleeping and dental hygiene. Talk to children and their parents about screen time when you see a child on any electronic device. Discuss choking hazards when the toddler is sitting in bed or in a chair eating.

Teach About Development

Ask team members to observe an infant or child, report on what the patient is able to do in each of the developmental domains, and then have them guess the patient's age. Ask trainees to compare what the patient before them can do versus what a child of this age should be able to do. Discuss how a child's development might be affected by their health condition and how observations about a child's development might be affected by the child's current experience in the hospital or clinic. As mentioned above, ask the trainees to compare patients: How do this child's language skills differ from the skills of the patient we just saw? Why?

Teach About Nutrition

Discuss appropriate (and inappropriate) nutrition in the context of what you observe the patient eating. With infants, talk about which types of foods would be the most appropriate to introduce next. Model ways to ask parents and children about what their typical diet is like and ways to incorporate nutritional suggestions in conversations with parents and patients.

Teach Broadly

Great clinical teachers broaden the teaching of medicine by discussing strategies to develop differential diagnosis,[5] limit cognitive bias,[6] and search for clinical answers in the literature.[7] They discuss sensitivity and specificity of laboratory results,[8] the cost of investigations,[9] and communication strategies.[10]

THINK OUT LOUD

Be explicit with your students; think out loud[11] and articulate how your clinical reasoning is changing as more information is learned. Great clinical teachers can explain how the components of the patient's history and physical examination lead them to make diagnoses. Examples of statements that could be articulated during an encounter with a child in respiratory distress include the following:

- Now that we've learned there is a positive history of asthma and eczema, I am more likely than before to think that this child has asthma.

- This child has audible wheezes. I am considering a diagnosis of a lower airway disease.

- The lack of wheezes doesn't rule out asthma in my mind; maybe this patient is not moving much air at all right now.

RECALL THE GREAT LEARNING

One of the most overlooked elements of bedside teaching is the necessity to reflect on the encounter.[12] A few minutes are needed to reflect on events during the encounter. Often students may not have noticed or appreciated specific events that can be brought to their attention. Feedback immediately after an encounter tends to be specific and thus more valuable.[13] Give students an opportunity to articulate simple learning goals that relate to the day's learning, such as looking up a clinical guideline or reviewing developmental milestones.

Remind trainees about the key learning acquired that day or ask them to keep a list of things they learned. In the midst of patient care, learners may be challenged to recall the teaching they experienced. Assess the session by requesting feedback and asking, "Next time we are at the bedside, should we do anything differently?" and "Did we achieve our goals for today?" Use this information to revise your future teaching sessions.

CONCLUSIONS

Medicine is learned at the bedside and each patient has a lesson to teach. In just a few minutes, great clinical teachers can direct students' attention to what is important while simultaneously providing clinical care. Timely teaching is a critical component of the tool kit of a great clinical teacher.

REFERENCES

1. Nagappan S, Hartsell A, Chandler N. Teaching in a family-centered care model: the exam room as the classroom. *Pediatrics.* 2013;131(5):836–838

2. Balighian E, Barone MA. Getting physical: the hypothesis driven physical exam. *Pediatrics.* 2016; 137(3):e20154511

3. Plant J, Barone MA, Serwint JR, Butani L. Taking humanism back to the bedside. *Pediatrics.* 2015;136(5): 828–830

4. Bannister SL, Hanson JL, Maloney CG, Dudas RA. Practical framework for fostering a positive learning environment. *Pediatrics.* 2015; 136(1):6–9

5. Bösner S, Pickert J, Stibane T. Teaching differential diagnosis in primary care using an inverted classroom approach: student satisfaction and gain in skills and knowledge. *BMC Med Educ.* 2015;15:63

6. Norman GR, Monteiro SD, Sherbino J, Ilgen JS, Schmidt HG, Mamede S. The causes of errors in clinical reasoning: cognitive biases, knowledge deficits, and dual process thinking. *Acad Med.* 2017;92(1):23–30

7. Sackett DL. Evidence-based medicine. *Semin Perinatol.* 1997;21(1):3–5

8. Smith BR, Aguero-Rosenfeld M, Anastasi J, et al; Academy of Clinical Laboratory Physicians and Scientists. Educating medical students in laboratory medicine: a proposed curriculum. *Am J Clin Pathol.* 2010;133(4):533–542

9. Aagaard E, Wagner R, Jackson D, Earnest M. Teaching the cost of hospital care to medical students. *MedEdPORTAL.* 2010;6:7787

10. Junod Perron N, Nendaz M, Louis-Simonet M, et al. Impact of postgraduate training on communication skills teaching: a controlled study. *BMC Med Educ.* 2014;14:80

11. Pinnock R, Young L, Spence F, Henning M, Hazell W. Can think aloud be used to teach and assess clinical reasoning in graduate medical education? *J Grad Med Educ.* 2015;7(3):334–337

12. Butani L, Blankenburg R, Long M. Stimulating reflective practice among your learners. *Pediatrics.* 2013;131(2):204–206

13. Gigante J, Dell M, Sharkey A. Getting beyond "good job": how to give effective feedback. *Pediatrics.* 2011;127(2):205–207

Getting Physical: The Hypothesis Driven Physical Exam

Eric Balighian, MD, Michael A. Barone, MD, MPH

The value of teaching at the patient's bedside has been recognized by generations of clinical teachers and students. In today's complex and fast-paced medical environment, clinical instructors teach at the bedside less frequently than in the past.[1,2] When learning the physical examination, medical students are often taught a series of 100+ anatomy-focused maneuvers.[3] The "head-to-toe" approach can help students practice complex maneuvers and develop an awareness of normal findings, but it has limitations in emphasizing the diagnostic relevance of the physical examination.[4] Teachers should guide students to transition from a head-to-toe physical examination to one used to support or refute potential diagnoses.

Emphasizing the physical examination's critical role in clinical reasoning can help to support improved diagnostic skills[5,6] and may lead to a cost conscious approach to testing. Numerous recommendations in the Choosing Wisely compendium highlight the critical role of the physical examination in high value care.[7] As part of the ongoing Council on Medical Student Education in Pediatrics series on skills used by great clinical teachers, this article introduces the Hypothesis Driven Physical Exam (HDPE).[5,6]

CONNECTING THE PHYSICAL EXAMINATION TO CLINICAL REASONING

An overview of clinical reasoning has been previously outlined in the series of articles from the Council on Medical Student Education in Pediatrics.[8] Perhaps the most important concept relevant to the physical examination is the search for, or anticipation of, specific findings identified from the history to confirm or exclude diagnoses. Experienced clinical teachers do this without conscious thought by activating stored medical knowledge. The sum of their learning and experience is bundled in the form of illness scripts: packaged information, which consists of memory points on mechanism, epidemiology, natural history, and clinical presentation of disease. Emphasizing how certain elements of the physical examination link to the "clinical presentation" or to other parts of an illness script is a fundamental element of teaching the HDPE.[9]

THE HDPE IN ACTION

Walking through a case can illustrate ways to emphasize the HDPE approach to clinical diagnosis.

A CASE

A 4-year-old boy is brought to clinic with a rash on his lower extremities. He is afebrile with

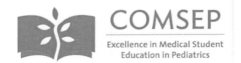

Department of Pediatrics, Johns Hopkins University School of Medicine, Baltimore, Maryland

DOI: 10.1542/peds.2015-4511

Accepted for publication Dec 14, 2015

Address correspondence to Michael A. Barone, MD, MPH, Johns Hopkins University School of Medicine, Charlotte Bloomberg Children's Hospital, 1800 Orleans St, Suite 8442, Baltimore, MD 21287. E-mail: mbarone@jhmi.edu

PEDIATRICS (ISSN Numbers: Print, 0031-4005; Online, 1098-4275).

FINANCIAL DISCLOSURE: The authors have indicated they have no financial relationships relevant to this article to disclose.

FUNDING: No external funding.

POTENTIAL CONFLICT OF INTEREST: The authors have indicated they have no potential conflicts of interest to disclose.

To cite: Balighian E and Barone MA. Getting Physical: The Hypothesis Driven Physical Exam. *Pediatrics.* 2016;137(3): e20154511

TABLE 1 Key Features of the Physical Examination

Diagnosis	Rash Characteristics and Distribution	Other Relevant Physical Findings
Immune thrombocytopenic purpura	Soft tissue bruising Numerous diffuse petechiae with scattered purpura	Oral mucosal bleeding Absent splenomegaly
Henoch-Schonlein purpura	Raised "palpable" petechiae with some coalescence to purpura, often from waist down	Abdominal tenderness Scrotal swelling Edema of the joint areas/extremities especially of the ankles and knees
Papular-purpuric gloves and stockings syndrome caused by parvovirus B19	Stocking and glove distribution of petechiae, often with sharp demarcation	Rash involves the genitalia and circumoral areas Cervical lymphadenopathy
Rickettsial disease	Acral distribution Macular/maculopapular component Palm and sole involvement Petechiae may be fewer in number	Child may appear unwell or have nuchal rigidity
Meningococcemia	Petechiae and purpura may be present, distribution often lower extremities if still well appearing	Child may appear unwell or mildly tachycardic
Leukemia or other hematologic malignancy	Nonspecific distribution of petechiae or purpura	Possible hepatosplenomegaly, mucosal bleeding, or lymphadenopathy

normal vital signs and is not ill appearing. The clinic nurse mentions to you the child seems to have petechiae on both legs. The student, preparing to see the patient, tells you she plans to ask questions about recent fever, illness, trauma, exposures, and travel, as well as the child's immunization history.

You quickly guide the student through a differential diagnosis of lower extremity petechiae in a well-appearing, afebrile child by using a HDPE framework. The differential diagnosis, limited for this example, would include immune thrombocytopenic purpura, Henoch-Schonlein purpura, and papular-purpuric gloves and stockings syndrome caused by parvovirus B19. You also caution the student not to miss a potentially devastating diagnosis such as rickettsial disease, meningococcemia, and leukemia. Thus, the key features of the physical examination would be useful to consider (Table 1).

PROMOTING AND INTEGRATING THE HDPE INTO DAILY PRACTICE: STRATEGIES

Direct Observation

You elect to join the student and directly observe her assess the patient.

TABLE 2 Script Sorting Grid

Red Eye	Preauricular Lymph Node	Bilateral	Purulent Exudate	Chemosis
Viral conjunctivitis	++	+	+/−	+
Bacterial conjunctivitis	—	—	++	++
Allergic conjunctivitis	—	++	−	+++

1. Ask the student for her initial differential diagnosis after she gathers the history but before she proceeds with the physical examination. When appropriate, explain this teaching moment respectfully to the patient and the parent at the bedside.

2. Guide the student toward physical examination findings, which help support or exclude possible diagnoses.

3. Observe the student performing the physical examination and give feedback on her physical examination skills.

4. Reconsider the differential diagnosis again, emphasizing how it may have changed after the examination.

5. Supplement the student's differential diagnosis with additional considerations if needed, and then demonstrate the examination features, which help to discriminate among the additional choices.

This strategy can also be used when listening to a student's clinical presentation. Prompts such as, "What physical findings, present or absent, could help you to differentiate among the diagnoses?" When doing this, try to then dedicate some time to reviewing the physical examination at the bedside.

Reviewing Notes

You read the student's note on the 4-year-old boy with petechiae. The note includes many nonrelevant findings that do not help support the student's assessment or plan.

1. Inform the student in advance that the physical examination sections of written notes are reviewed for diagnostic relevance and reasoning.

2. Review the note with specific attention to:

   o The student's documentation of relevant parts of the examination. For example, a detailed description of the distribution of the petechiae

   o Negative findings of importance. For example, lack of splenomegaly.

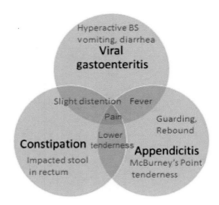

FIGURE 1
Abdominal pain.

- o A patient's assessment and differential diagnosis supported by the physical examination.

3. Guide the student through making connections between physical findings and the diagnostic possibilities.

4. Follow-up with review of subsequent notes for improvement.

Small Group Teaching

You decide to discuss the case of the child with petechiae the following day with multiple students in a case-based learning session. One student presents the patient's history and then you facilitate a discussion.

1. Ask each student to list a limited number of important features they would seek on the patient's physical examination. "Based on the patient's history thus far, and our working differential diagnosis, what are 3 or 4 specific findings you would look for on the patient's physical exam?" (eg, palpable petechiae, splenomegaly, mucosal lesions, joint swelling).

2. Guide the students further: "How would each physical finding, or lack of the finding, support your diagnostic hypotheses?"

Additional Learning Exercises

Emphasizing the physical examination's role in clinical reasoning can also be accomplished by assigning students brief learning exercises before or after a patient encounter or clinic session. Examples of such exercises include script sorting and the use of visual Venn diagrams.[9] These exercises can be completed by the student during a prescribed amount of time (overnight, before the next clinical session or patient, etc.) and can then be reviewed with a preceptor.

Script Sorting

Script sorting allows students to assign a weight or priority to certain competing diagnoses on the basis of elements of the history or, as in this example, the physical examination of a child with a red eye. The teacher and/or the student create the grid for the student to complete (Table 2).

Visual Venn Diagrams

A visual representation of the diagnostic possibilities can be an effective teaching method. Students are asked to contribute common or shared features (in areas where circles overlap) and should prioritize eliciting findings that are specific or differentiating (nonoverlapping areas). An example is presented for abdominal pain (Fig 1).

CONCLUSIONS

The HDPE can be used on a daily basis and need not be a time-intensive teaching strategy. Learning the physical examination in a rote head-to-toe manner may be an effective early learning strategy for students, but the physical examination's clinical utility will be increased if driven by diagnostic hypotheses. The HDPE can be a stimulus to return to bedside teaching. Furthermore, the great clinical teacher can emphasize the role of the physical examination, putting focus on the important concepts of clinical reasoning and high value care.

ABBREVIATION

HDPE: Hypothesis Driven Physical Exam

REFERENCES

1. Crumlish CM, Yialamas MA, McMahon GT. Quantification of bedside teaching by an academic hospitalist group. *J Hosp Med.* 2009;4(5):304–307

2. LaCombe MA. On bedside teaching. *Ann Intern Med.* 1997;126(3):217–220

3. Yudkowsky R, Downing S, Klamen D, Valaski M, Eulenberg B, Popa M. Assessing the head-to-toe physical examination skills of medical students. *Med Teach.* 2004;26(5):415–419

4. Yudkowsky R, Otaki J, Lowenstein T, Riddle J, Nishigori H, Bordage G. A hypothesis-driven physical examination learning and assessment procedure for medical students: initial validity evidence. *Med Educ.* 2009;43(8):729–740

5. Yudkowsky R, Otaki J, Bordage G, Lowenstein T, Riddle J, Nishigori H. Hypothesis-driven physical examination student handbook. MedEdPORTAL Publications; 2011. Available at: https://www.mededportal.org/publication/8294. Accessed December 14, 2015

6. Nishigori H, Masuda K, Kikukawa M, et al. A model teaching session for the hypothesis-driven physical examination. *Med Teach.* 2011;33(5):410–417

7. Choosing Wisely Master List. ABIM Foundation. Available at: www.choosingwisely.org/clinician-lists/. Accessed October 2, 2015

8. Fleming A, Cutrer W, Reimschisel T, Gigante J. You too can teach clinical reasoning! *Pediatrics.* 2012;130(5):795–797

9. Stuart E, Slavin S, Butani L, Blankenburg R, Konopasek L. Clinical reasoning. In: Morgenstern B, ed. *Guidebook for Clerkship Directors,* Chapter 8. North Syracuse, NY: Gegensatz Press; 2012

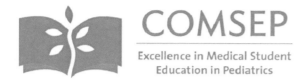

AUTHORS: Suresh Nagappan, MD, MSPH, Angela Hartsell, MD, MPH, and Nicole Chandler, MD

Cone Health Pediatrics, Department of Pediatrics, University of North Carolina, Greensboro, North Carolina

Address correspondence to Suresh Nagappan, MD, MSPH, Cone Health Pediatrics, Department of Pediatrics, University of North Carolina, 1200 North Elm St, Greensboro, NC 27401. E-mail: suresh.nagappan@conehealth.com

Accepted for publication Feb 13, 2013

ABBREVIATIONS
FCC—family-centered care
FCR—family-centered rounds

doi:10.1542/peds.2013-0489

Teaching in a Family-Centered Care Model: The Exam Room as the Classroom

"To study the phenomenon of disease without books is to sail an uncharted sea, while to study books without patients is not to go to sea at all."
Sir William Osler, 1903

Although Osler challenges us to study disease in the context of patients, family-centered care (FCC) challenges us to study disease in front of and alongside our patients. This article focuses on teaching in the presence of patients and families, at the bedside and during outpatient encounters, as part of the ongoing Council on Medical Student Education in Pediatrics series on skills and strategies used by superb clinical teachers.

WHAT IS FCC?

FCC is rooted in collaboration among patients, families, physicians (including those in training), and nurses.[1] It is guided by the principles of respecting the patient and family, building on each family's strengths, being flexible, offering choices about care when possible, being transparent, and collaborating with families to make shared decisions.[1] Long before the term was coined in the second half of the 20th century, FCC was practiced by many pediatricians and family physicians.

FCC in practice has decreased length of stay and readmission rates,[2] but benefits to learners have been less well documented. FCC is difficult to teach in a traditional classroom setting and is better demonstrated though role modeling and including learners in the partnership of care. One method of incorporating FCC into teaching is through family-centered rounds (FCR) or family-centered discussions both at the bedside and in the examination room.

Sisterhen et al[3] defined FCR as "interdisciplinary work rounds at the bedside in which the patient and family share in the control of the management plan as well as in the evaluation of the process itself." FCC with FCR provides an opportunity for learners to observe attending physicians' bedside manner, physical examination techniques, and interactions with patients in both inpatient and outpatient settings. Preceptors can also directly observe students taking histories, examining patients, and counseling children and families, all of which are more effectively taught in the presence of a patient. By teaching at the bedside in the context of a real patient, students are more likely to receive immediate,

relevant knowledge that will "stick with" them. Having role models who teach, and learn, in front of patients assists students in developing their own communication skills and bedside manner.[4]

IN THE CLINIC

A common concern of busy preceptors is finding the time to teach while running a hectic clinic. A study by Baker et al[5] in the clinic setting found that examination room presentations (in which the student presents the case in front of the patient, family, and preceptor in the examination room rather than to the preceptor alone outside the examination room) took a similar amount of time and resulted in higher patient satisfaction than conference room presentations. Anderson et al[6] showed that clinic patients who experienced examination room presentations by learners preferred this method when offered a choice for future visits.

Teaching in an FCC environment also affords preceptors an opportunity to role model, and teach, different styles of communication. Although it is difficult to explain to a student how to be empathic or reassure a worried parent or discuss a complex medical problem, it is possible to demonstrate these skills by talking to patients and families in the presence of students. In a 2008 focus group by Williams et al,[7] a medical student stated, "It's very powerful if you see the example on an actual person, and especially if you know more about their story, their background, you're more likely to take something away from that experience, whether it be some kernel of knowledge about a disease or a certain way of interacting with patients." The family and the patient, when approached with respect, become an integral part of the teaching process.

ON INPATIENT ROUNDS

Teaching in an FCC environment is beneficial in the inpatient setting as well. A 2003 American Academy of Pediatrics policy statement recommended that FCR be standard practice.[8] Since then, FCR has become the predominant method by which inpatient rounds are conducted on pediatric wards around the country.[9] Although Muething et al[10] found that it took 20% longer for FCR in the inpatient setting, there were other time savings downstream, such as less frequent call backs to answer questions from families or nurses. With FCR, the student has the opportunity to practice effective ways of communicating with families by using understandable language, avoiding jargon, and involving families in the decision-making process.

LEARNERS' PERSPECTIVES

Learners, though, are not convinced. Although 85% of patients prefer presentations in their rooms, only 53% of learners think that presenting in the presence of the family is more educational than conference room rounding.[11] In a randomized controlled trial,

learners were significantly more comfortable asking questions (84% vs 69%) and being asked questions (85% vs 67%) when presenting in the conference room; only 4% of students felt comfortable presenting in front of families.[12] Wang-Cheng et al,[13] in a 1989 survey, found that 95% of residents preferred to do presentations away from the patient. Many reported a fear of looking foolish in front of a parent. This fear is especially acute in students, many of whom are struggling to develop their basic presentation skills.

The additional task of trying to maintain rapport with families leads to added discomfort. In a focus group on FCR of students from the University of North Carolina rotating at Cone Health, a medical student noted, "I think it's very hard to earn the respect of the patients and family as a student. I think giving constructive feedback to junior members of the team is easily and often misconstrued by families as a lack of confidence in those team members, which consequently makes it hard for families to trust their judgment." Although these concerns are valid, students do become more comfortable presenting in front of patients with practice and experience in FCR.[10,14] In Cox et al's[14] survey of medical students who had completed a 6-week pediatric clerkship that included presenting in front of patients, only 17% were concerned about being "pimped." Many come to believe that teaching is more relevant during FCR and that they learn in ways that are not practical in the conference room.[10,15]

TIPS FOR TEACHERS

For FCR to succeed as an educational tool, these legitimate learner concerns need to be addressed. A resident in Williams et al's[7] focus group stated, "If teachers can set the tone and what the expectations are and say that 'it is

okay to make mistakes, we all make mistakes, but the great doctors are the ones who take those mistakes and use them to improve themselves,' that's the best way to learn in that stressful environment." The preceptor can set the tone for a safe learning environment with the following practical steps:

- Set expectations at the beginning of the learner's rotation.
- Introduce the members of the health care team and acknowledge their level of training.
- Acknowledge to the learner the stress of presenting in front of patients and families along with the preceptor's goal of supporting the learner without humiliation.
- Give the learner permission to "not know" and ask for help.
- If a learner says something incorrectly or inappropriately, use positive reinforcement to acknowledge what was correct and then explain what the actual plan will be.
- Offer direct constructive feedback outside the patient's room.[4]
- Direct Socratic questioning to the group instead of an individual whenever possible.

Teaching in an FCC environment does, however, have limitations. Some important discussions, such as reviewing extensive differential diagnoses or considering highly sensitive topics, such as abuse, may be better held outside the patient's room.

CONCLUSIONS

FCR in both inpatient and outpatient settings benefits patients and learners. It has the potential to assist in creating a supportive environment in which trainees learn by watching and listening to their attending physicians, by making mistakes and correcting them, and by connecting with patients and families.

ACKNOWLEDGMENTS

We gratefully acknowledge Drs Janice Hanson, Robert Dudas, and Susan Bannister for their extensive comments and editing.

REFERENCES

1. Committee on Hospital Care and Institute for Patient- and Family-Centered Care. Patient- and family-centered care and the pediatrician's role. *Pediatrics*. 2012;129(2): 394–404

2. Forsythe P. New practices in the transitional care center improve outcomes for babies and their families. *J Perinatol*. 1998; 18(6 pt 2 suppl):S13–S17

3. Sisterhen LL, Blaszak RT, Woods MB, Smith CE. Defining family-centered rounds. *Teach Learn Med*. 2007;19(3):319–322

4. Young HN, Schumacher JB, Moreno MA, et al. Medical student self-efficacy with family-centered care during bedside rounds. *Acad Med*. 2012;87(6):767–775

5. Baker RC, Klein M, Samaan Z, Brinkman W. Exam room presentations and teaching in outpatient pediatrics: effects on visit duration and parent, attending physician, and resident perceptions. *Ambul Pediatr*. 2007;7 (5):354–359

6. Anderson RJ, Cyran E, Schilling L, et al. Outpatient case presentations in the conference room versus examination room: results from two randomized controlled trials. *Am J Med*. 2002;113(8):657–662

7. Williams KN, Ramani S, Fraser B, Orlander JD. Improving bedside teaching: findings from a focus group study of learners. *Acad Med*. 2008;83(3):257–264

8. Committee on Hospital Care. American Academy of Pediatrics. Family-centered care and the pediatrician's role. *Pediatrics*. 2003;112(3 pt 1):691–697

9. Mittal VS, Sigrest T, Ottolini MC, et al. Family-centered rounds on pediatric wards: a PRIS network survey of US and Canadian hospitalists. *Pediatrics*. 2010;126(1):37–43

10. Muething SE, Kotagal UR, Schoettker PJ, Gonzalez del Rey J, DeWitt TG. Family-centered bedside rounds: a new approach to patient care and teaching. *Pediatrics*. 2007;119(4): 829–832

11. Gonzalo JD, Chuang CH, Huang G, Smith C. The return of bedside rounds: an educational intervention. *J Gen Intern Med*. 2010; 25(8):792–798

12. Landry MA, Lafrenaye S, Roy MC, Cyr CA. A randomized, controlled trial of bedside versus conference-room case presentation in a pediatric intensive care unit. *Pediatrics*. 2007;120(2):275–280

13. Wang-Cheng RM, Barnas GP, Sigmann P, Riendl PA, Young MJ. Bedside case presentations: why patients like them but learners don't. *J Gen Intern Med*. 1989;4(4): 284–287

14. Cox ED, Schumacher JB, Young HN, Evans MD, Moreno MA, Sigrest TD. Medical student outcomes after family-centered bedside rounds. *Acad Pediatr*. 2011;11(5):403–408

15. Chauke HL, Pattinson RC. Ward rounds—bedside or conference room? *S Afr Med J*. 2006;96(5):398–400

FINANCIAL DISCLOSURE: *The authors have indicated they have no financial relationships relevant to this article to disclose.*
FUNDING: No external funding.

The Whole "PROOF": Incorporating Evidence-Based Medicine Into Clinical Teaching

Nicholas M. Potisek, MD,[a] Kenya McNeal-Trice, MD,[b] Michael A. Barone, MD, MPH[c]

As part of the ongoing Council on Medical Student Education in Pediatrics series on skills used by great clinical teachers, this article introduces teaching strategies to more effectively convey the principles of evidence-based medicine (EBM), including a mnemonic that can serve as a framework for clinician educators.

EBM is the selective use of best current evidence to make medical decisions for individual patients.[1] Incorporating medical evidence into clinical practice is an expectation for medical students entering residency.[2] Routinely practicing EBM can promote patient safety, improve quality, and enhance value in health care.[3] Resources exist for faculty to review the basic tenets of EBM.[4]

To ensure students entering residency have a strong foundation in EBM, clinical teachers need to teach EBM while providing patient care. Many interventions developed to improve teaching of critical appraisal skills are applicable to the classroom but not at the patient's bedside.[5,6] Clinician educators need to know how to guide trainees through the process of establishing answerable clinical questions, appraising evidence, and applying evidence to patient care.

Clinical educators are faced with several challenges to teaching EBM, such as lack of time and a paucity of EBM curriculum requirements.[7] Learning EBM is difficult because students may lack clinical role models, wrestle with acknowledging uncertainty, and struggle with applying evidence to patient care.[8] If barriers are not addressed, an inability to incorporate EBM into patient care can persist into residency training and beyond.[9]

The key elements of EBM can be summarized by using the mnemonic PROOF (Table 1): Propose a clinical question, review the literature, organize and appraise literature search results, overlap evidence and specific patient care needs and values, and follow patient outcomes. The following clinical scenario helps illustrate how to use PROOF in a clinical teaching setting.

A 6-year-old girl with mild persistent asthma presents for a follow-up visit 3 days after treatment in an emergency department (ED). Review of the ED visit reveals that β-agonists and a single dose of dexamethasone led to the patient's clinical improvement and her discharge from the ED. Today, before entering the clinic room to see the patient, your medical student asks, "Can a single dose of dexamethasone be used to reduce hospitalization? I've primarily seen a 5-day course of prednisone used."

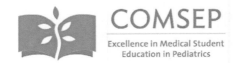

[a]Department of Pediatrics, Wake Forest Baptist Medical Center, Winston-Salem, North Carolina; [b]Division of General Pediatrics and Adolescent Medicine, North Carolina Children's Hospital, Chapel Hill, North Carolina; and [c]Department of Pediatrics, Johns Hopkins University School of Medicine, Baltimore, Maryland

Drs Potisek and Barone conceptualized, designed, and drafted the initial manuscript; Dr McNeal-Trice drafted the initial manuscript; and all authors revised the manuscript and approved the final manuscript as submitted.

DOI: https://doi.org/10.1542/peds.2017-1073

Accepted for publication Mar 29, 2017

Address correspondence to Nicholas M. Potisek, MD, Department of Pediatrics, Wake Forest School of Medicine, Medical Center Blvd, Winston-Salem, NC 27157. E-mail: npotisek@wakehealth.edu

PEDIATRICS (ISSN Numbers: Print, 0031-4005; Online, 1098-4275).

FINANCIAL DISCLOSURE: The authors have indicated they have no financial relationships relevant to this article to disclose.

FUNDING: No external funding.

POTENTIAL CONFLICT OF INTEREST: The authors have indicated they have no potential conflicts of interest to disclose.

To cite: Potisek NM, McNeal-Trice K, Barone MA. The Whole "PROOF": Incorporating Evidence-Based Medicine Into Clinical Teaching. *Pediatrics*. 2017;140(1):e20171073

TABLE 1 PROOF Strategies

Key EBM Elements	Clinical Strategies
Propose a clinical question	Guide PICO-formatted questions
	What is the question we are trying to answer?
	Can this question be framed into PICO format?
	If you designed a study to answer this question, what patient population would you study?
	Any specific inclusion or exclusion criteria to consider?
	Select topics for learners with sufficient evidence to explore
Review the literature	Identify specific systematic reviews, guidelines, or research articles for learners
	Review references from articles, reviews
	Introduce Cochrane database or *BMJ Clinical Evidence*
	Have team member demonstrate search strategy
	Incorporate medical librarians and informationists
Organize and appraise search results	Ensure leaners know hierarchy of evidence
	Have learners focus on specific aspects of critical appraisal (internal and external validity, number needed to treat, likelihood ratios)
Overlap evidence and specific patient care needs and values	Guide questions to ensure care is patient specific
	Is this patient similar to those included in the study?
	Do our treatment options meet our patient's values?
	Use *JAMA* series "Users' Guides to the Medical Literature"
Follow patient outcomes	Debrief patient outcomes
	Emphasize use of medical literature in decision making during patient encounters
	Role model and acknowledge challenges by using EBM in various clinical situations

PROPOSE A CLINICAL QUESTION

Formulating a clinical question is essential to the practice of EBM. Clinical educators can model how to develop clinical questions during routine delivery of patient care. Learners can be guided through intentional questions to characterize the patient population, intervention, comparison, and desired outcome (PICO),[10] such as "What is the clinical question we are trying to answer for this patient?" or "If you were designing a study to answer this clinical question, what patients would you want to include?" Instead of referencing a specific article, learners can benefit when a clinical educator helps facilitate question framing by selecting topics with sufficient evidence available to explore. Clinical questions structured in the PICO format can improve search results.[11] In our example, the question posed by the student can be framed into the following PICO-style clinical question: "Are children with an acute asthma exacerbation [patient population] who receive dexamethasone [intervention] instead of 5 days of prednisone [comparison] less likely to be admitted to the hospital [outcome]?"

REVIEW THE LITERATURE

Clinical educators can guide learners to specific, relevant systematic reviews, guidelines, or research articles. References from these evidence summaries can be used to identify appropriate articles. Learners can be pointed to the Cochrane Database of Systematic Reviews or *BMJ Clinical Evidence* to jump-start their searches.[12,13] When conducting evidence searches, the learner can demonstrate his or her search strategy to the team. Clinical educators can then demonstrate their own search strategies and compare them to the learner's strategies and results. Incorporating the expertise of medical librarians and informationists can promote interprofessional collaboration and assist when clinical demands limit time to perform searching. Informationists are clinical librarians with specific training in information-seeking skills and knowledge in a given specialty area. Literature searches can be made more efficient by using appropriate filters and/or limits, display settings, full-text icons, clinical queries, medical subject headings, and related citations. In our example, the clinical educator could specifically ask the student to find a recent 2014 systematic review published in *Pediatrics* to help start the search and then view related citations.[14]

ORGANIZE AND APPRAISE LITERATURE SEARCH RESULTS

Appraisal of the literature remains a challenge to teach while providing clinical care because of time constraints. An initial first step is ensuring students learn the hierarchy of evidence. Randomized controlled trials represent the highest quality evidence, followed by observational studies, case reports, and finally, expert opinion. Structured formats to appraise articles should be made available to learners. Among the most well-known is *The Journal of the American Medical Association* (*JAMA*) series entitled "Users' Guides to the Medical Literature."[15,16] Great clinical educators encourage a structured critical analysis of the literature, and these resources provide students with a logical framework. When teaching critical appraisal techniques, it is essential not to overload the learners. For example, if a learner is reviewing an article for the team, have him or her focus on 1 aspect of critical appraisal. In our example, the student could be asked to review how to interpret the forest plots included in the systematic review.

OVERLAP EVIDENCE AND SPECIFIC PATIENT CARE NEEDS AND VALUES

Emphasizing the importance of using evidence to meet specific patient needs is a critical step in the successful implementation of clinical EBM. The question "Is this patient similar to those included in the study?" can demonstrate the application of evidence to a specific patient. It is often useful to point out the limitations of studies generalized to a specific patient's care, highlight the ambiguity of medicine, and have learners observe your discussion with the patient and the patient's family about such ambiguity. Resources to help match evidence with specific patient care needs and values include the *JAMA* series and a manual for evidence-based clinical practice.[15,17] In our example, the clinical educator could ask the student to assess either the severity of asthma among patients included in the systematic review or the dose of dexamethasone provided.

FOLLOW PATIENT OUTCOMES

Finally, following a patient's response to an EBM-guided test or treatment validates the relevance of EBM for learners. Intentionally debriefing patient outcomes of EBM decisions allows each learner to explore context and generalizability to future clinical practice. When communicating with patients and families, clinical educators should model the emphasis on how the medical literature was used to guide diagnostic or treatment decisions. In our example, one could encourage the student to call the patient's caretakers a few days after the EBM-guided decision to assess continued recovery or any additional unscheduled care. Skilled clinicians acknowledge the difficulty of balancing available evidence, anecdotal experiences, and individual patient preferences when making clinical decisions. Transparency in a clinician's thought process helps learners refine their clinical decision-making and creates a safe environment to discuss appropriate use of EBM.

CONCLUSIONS

Great educators understand that teaching clinical skills such as diagnostic reasoning and performing physical examinations can be enhanced

through the use of frameworks. The same is true for EBM. PROOF can assist all team members in learning the necessary steps for proposing and answering clinical questions through use of the medical literature. Learners want PROOF that evidence-based care can benefit patients.

ABBREVIATIONS

EBM: evidence-based medicine
ED: emergency department
JAMA: *The Journal of the American Medical Association*
PICO: patient, intervention, comparison, and outcome
PROOF: propose, review, organize, overlap, and follow

REFERENCES

1. Sackett DL, Rosenberg WM, Gray JA, Haynes RB, Richardson WS. Evidence based medicine: what it is and what it isn't. *BMJ*. 1996;312(7023):71–72

2. Association of American Medical Colleges. Core entrustable professional activities for entering residency (updated). Available at: www.mededportal.org/icollaborative/resource/887. Accessed March 20, 2016

3. Medicine IoMRoE-B. *Institute of Medicine: Roundtable on Evidence-Based Medicine*. Washington, DC: National Academy of Sciences; 2009

4. Isenburg MV. LibGuides: evidence-based practice. http://guides.mclibrary.duke.edu/ebm. Accessed October 26, 2016

5. Maggio LA, Tannery NH, Chen HC, ten Cate O, O'Brien B. Evidence-based medicine training in undergraduate medical education: a review and critique of the literature published 2006-2011. *Acad Med*. 2013;88(7):1022–1028

6. Tilson JK, Kaplan SL, Harris JL, et al. Sicily statement on classification and development of evidence-based practice learning assessment tools. *BMC Med Educ*. 2011;11:78

7. Oude Rengerink K, Thangaratinam S, Barnfield G, et al. How can we teach

EBM in clinical practice? An analysis of barriers to implementation of on-the-job EBM teaching and learning. *Med Teach*. 2011;33(3):e125–e130

8. Maggio LA, ten Cate O, Chen HC, Irby DM, O'Brien BC. Challenges to learning evidence-based medicine and educational approaches to meet these challenges: a qualitative study of selected EBM curricula in U.S. and Canadian Medical Schools. *Acad Med*. 2016;91(1):101–106

9. Green ML, Ruff TR. Why do residents fail to answer their clinical questions? A qualitative study of barriers to practicing evidence-based medicine. *Acad Med*. 2005;80(2):176–182

10. Richardson WS, Wilson MC, Nishikawa J, Hayward RS. The well-built clinical question: a key to evidence-based decisions. *ACP J Club*. 1995;123(3):A12–A13

11. Schardt C, Adams MB, Owens T, Keitz S, Fontelo P. Utilization of the PICO framework to improve searching PubMed for clinical questions. *BMC Med Inform Decis Mak*. 2007;7:16

12. Cochrane, John Wiley & Sons. Cochrane Library. Available at: www.cochranelibrary.com/. Accessed 2016

13. BMJ Publishing Group. Welcome to *BMJ Clinical Evidence*. Available at: http://clinicalevidence.bmj.com/x/index.html. Accessed October 26, 2016

14. Keeney GE, Gray MP, Morrison AK, et al. Dexamethasone for acute asthma exacerbations in children: a meta-analysis. *Pediatrics*. 2014;133(3):493–499

15. Guyatt GH, Sackett DL, Cook DJ. Users' guides to the medical literature. II. How to use an article about therapy or prevention. A. Are the results of the study valid? Evidence-Based Medicine Working Group. *JAMA*. 1993;270(21):2598–2601

16. Jaeschke R, Guyatt G, Sackett DL. Users' guides to the medical literature. III. How to use an article about a diagnostic test. A. Are the results of the study valid? Evidence-Based Medicine Working Group. *JAMA*. 1994;271(5):389–391

17. Guyatt G, Rennie D, Meade M, Cook D; American Medical Association. *Users' Guides to the Medical Literature. A Manual for Evidence-Based Clinical Practice*. 3rd ed. New York, NY: McGraw-Hill Education Medical; 2015

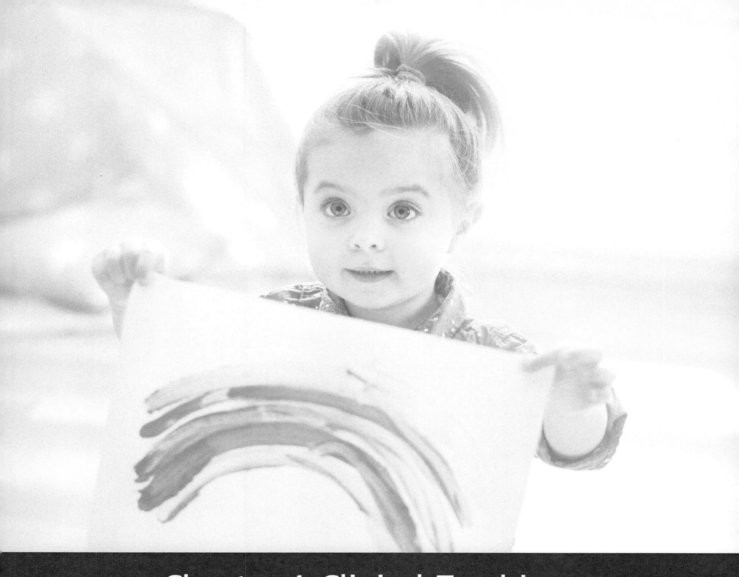

Chapter 4: Clinical Teaching

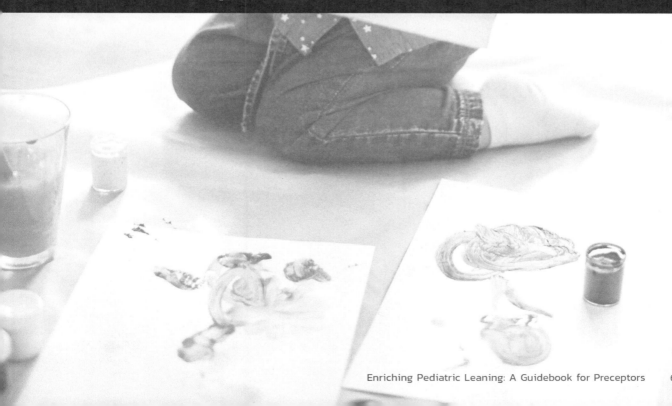

Chapter 4

The Heart Of Clinical Teaching: Observation, Feedback, Assessment, And Evaluation

By Janice L Hanson, PhD, EdS, MH
Professor of Medicine, Washington University in St. Louis

Observation and feedback in clinical learning environments are central tenets of medical education. Almost 4 decades ago, Ende published a landmark paper that described best practices in feedback that we still use today.[1] At that time, medical students and residents received little direct observation of their performance in clinical settings and very little feedback about the quality and accuracy of their work. Ende articulated that clinical learners need formative feedback to help them progress and described a model for preceptors. He emphasized that effective feedback begins by observing learners working in the clinical environment, focusing on specific behaviors, and providing recommendations for improvement. He suggested that teachers and learners work as allies toward common goals. Ende acknowledged the importance of evaluation as a summative judgment about how well a learner had met a particular goal; but first, all learners need opportunities to work toward a goal and receive formative feedback before a teacher reaches conclusions about their performance.

The 6 articles in this chapter build on the core features of observation, feedback, assessment, and evaluation that Ende described, providing practical tips for clinical teachers. "Oh, What You Can See" reviews the advantages of direct observation and provides suggestions for ensuring that observation happens in busy clinical settings.[2] While finding time to directly observe medical students and residents is a continuing challenge, Lane and Gottlieb remind us in their article about structured clinical observations that it takes just 3–5 minutes of observation to see enough of a learner's clinical skills to formulate feedback.[3] Focusing on a learner's skills in history taking or physical examinations or giving information to patients and families helps make observation feasible in the busy clinical environment. In the second article, Gigante et al explain that these few minutes of observation provide the foundation for effective feedback.[4] They reinforce the importance of going beyond general compliments to pointing out specific behaviors and guidance for improvement. They differentiate between brief, daily feedback and major feedback, which may occur weekly or at the midpoint of a rotation—and they remind us that brief, daily feedback takes minimal time in the clinical setting but nevertheless makes a noticeable difference in learning clinical skills.[5]

The third and fourth articles in this chapter encourage teachers to look more deeply at the needs of learners when teaching in clinical settings. Bernstein et al address how to "diagnose the learner in difficulty."[6] This involves listening and observing the learner in more detail, diagnosing the learner's needs, then developing, documenting, and communicating a specific plan to help the learner improve. Hanson et al detail how to make assessments "in the moment" while teaching, to tailor teaching to the needs of individual learners.[7] This article reminds clinical teachers to elicit goals, which hearkens back to Ende's point that teachers and learners should work as allies toward common goals. This article provides clear examples of useful strategies for assessing while teaching, while adding minimal extra time to the teacher's day.

These articles all emphasize the importance of a framework for observation and feedback, a lens to help the clinical teacher focus on the performance of the student, make a relevant assessment about the learner's progress toward clinical skill, and provide targeted feedback and evaluation. "Assessment for Learning" explains how to use the RIME (Reporter, Interpreter, Manager, and Educator) framework as this lens. Dr. Louis Pangaro developed the RIME framework in the 1980s and 1990s while teaching medical students and guiding faculty toward effective teaching and assessment, first publishing about RIME in 1999.[8] RIME functions follow the familiar rhythm of caring for patients. When filling the reporter function, a learner gathers and presents observations; as an interpreter, the learner makes an assessment of what the data about a patient means; as a manager/educator, the learner develops a plan for managing the patient's care and educates the patient, themself, and others about this plan.[8-10] Thinking about a learner's clinical skills in these 4 categories can assist a teacher in describing a plan to help the learner progress and grow as a physician.

The fifth article in the chapter provides guidance for summative feedback, with practical tips for writing comments for evaluations.[11] This article also applies the RIME framework, outlining a way to structure written comments about a student's performance during a rotation. The authors add 2 practical tips to the RIME framework: (1) Add a P to remind teachers to include comments on professionalism; and (2) Add a specific recommendation for improvement and development. The resulting PRIME+ title helps preceptors remember the key elements to include when writing narrative evaluations.

The last article in the chapter brings the sequence of observation, feedback, assessment, and evaluation to a culmination in writing a letter of recommendation for a student's application to residency.[12] Devon et al remind us of the importance of the words we use to describe a student, and of focusing on the goals and strengths of each individual. The letter of recommendation provides an opportunity to tell the story of a student's educational trajectory and professional potential, with assessment and evaluation providing the illustrations that bring the student's story to life.

Taken together, these articles describe the rhythm of teaching for the clinical teacher: observe the learner, assess the learner, provide feedback to promote learning, and repeat this pattern of observation, assessment, and feedback to support the learner in accomplishing goals toward improved clinical skills.[9,13] This pattern of teaching mirrors the rhythm of clinical care—listen to and observe a patient, gather more data, make an assessment, develop a plan— or SOAP: symptoms, observations, assessment, and plan.[14] After teaching in this way, the preceptor is in a good position to write summative feedback. After a short time with a learner, the teacher can write about brief observations and feedback. After several days or weeks with a learner, a teacher will have completed enough observations and feedback to write a more comprehensive evaluation or a letter of recommendation—one that includes specific examples of the care the learner has provided, clear guidance for future learning and development as a physician, and evaluative statements about the learner's progress toward their goals.[9]

The rhythm of assessment and feedback forms the heart of clinical teaching, passing the practice of medicine from teacher to learner. The articles in this chapter provide a wonderful collection of practical advice for honing these skills.

References

1. Ende J. Feedback in clinical medical education. *JAMA*. 1983;250(6):777-781.
2. Hanson JL, Bannister SL, Clark A, Raszka WV, Jr. Oh, what you can see: the role of observation in medical student education. *Pediatrics*. 2010;126(5):843-845.
3. Lane JL, Gottlieb RP. Structured clinical observations: a method to teach clinical skills with limited time and financial resources. *Pediatrics*. 2000;105(4 Pt 2):973-977.
4. Gigante J, Dell M, Sharkey A. Getting beyond "Good job": how to give effective feedback. *Pediatrics*. 2011;127(2):205-207.
5. Branch WT, Jr., Paranjape A. Feedback and reflection: teaching methods for clinical settings. *Acad Med*. 2002;77(12 Pt 1):1185-1188.
6. Bernstein S, Atkinson AR, Martimianakis MA. Diagnosing the learner in difficulty. *Pediatrics*. 2013;132(2):210-212.
7. Hanson JL, Wallace CM, Bannister SL. Assessment for Learning: How to Assess Your Learners' Performance in the Clinical Environment. *Pediatrics*. 2020;145(3).
8. Pangaro L. A new vocabulary and other innovations for improving descriptive in-training evaluations. *Acad Med*. 1999;74(11):1203-1207.
9. Pangaro LN. A primer of evaluation terminology: Definitions and important distinctions in evaluation. In: Pangaro LN, McGaghie WC, eds. *Handbook on Medical Student Evaluation and Assessment*. North Syracuse, New York: Gegensatz Press; 2015.
10. Stephens MB, Gimbel RW, Pangaro L. Commentary: The RIME/EMR scheme: an educational approach to clinical documentation in electronic medical records. *Acad Med*. 2011;86(1):11-14.
11. Holmes AV, Peltier CB, Hanson JL, Lopreiato JO. Writing medical student and resident performance evaluations: beyond "performed as expected". *Pediatrics*. 2014;133(5):766-768.
12. Devon EP, Burns R, Hartke A. The LETTER of recommendation: Showcasing a student's strengths. *Pediatrics*. **NEED TO INSERT CITATION DETAILS – NOT PUBLISHED YET**
13. Pangaro LN. Why Isn't a Diagnosis Deep Enough? A Perspective from Internal Medicine. Artiss Symposium 2016: Understanding the Patients' Experiences: Beyond Diagnostic Labels; 2016; Bethesda, Maryland.
14. Podder V, Lew V, Ghassemzadeh S. SOAP Notes. [Updated 2020 Sep 3]. *StatPearls [Internet]*. 2020(January). https://www.ncbi.nlm.nih.gov/books/NBK482263/. Accessed 12/14/20.

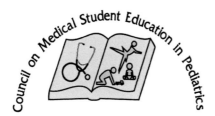

CONTRIBUTORS: Janice L. Hanson, PhD, EdS,[a] Susan L. Bannister, MD,[b] Alexandra Clark, MD,[c] and William V. Raszka Jr, MD[d]

[a]Departments of Medicine and Pediatrics, Uniformed Services University of the Health Sciences, Bethesda, Maryland; [b]Department of Pediatrics, Faculty of Medicine, University of Calgary, Calgary, Alberta, Canada; [c]Department of Pediatrics, Loma Linda University School of Medicine, Loma Linda, CA; and [d]Department of Pediatrics, University of Vermont College of Medicine, Burlington, Vermont

Address correspondence to Janice L. Hanson, PhD, EdS, Departments of Medicine and Pediatrics, Uniformed Services University of the Health Sciences, 4301 Jones Bridge Rd, Bethesda, MD 20814. E-mail: jhanson@usuhs.edu

Accepted for publication Aug 24, 2010

The views expressed are those of the authors and not necessarily those of the Uniformed Services University or the Department of Defense.

doi:10.1542/peds.2010-2538

Oh, What You Can See: The Role of Observation in Medical Student Education

This article is the third in a series by the Council on Medical Student Education in Pediatrics (COMSEP) that focuses on skills and strategies that can help good clinical teachers become great. The purpose of this article is to outline the critical role of observation in medical student education settings. Observation of students can take many forms, including direct observation during a clinical encounter (eg, taking a history, performing a physical examination, or talking with patients and families), with a standardized patient, or indirectly while watching a videotaped encounter. In this article, we focus on direct observation of medical students in clinical settings for the purpose of gathering information for feedback and student assessment.

BACKGROUND In the past 2 decades, medical education has shifted toward competency-based curricula in which students must demonstrate specific skills and behaviors.[1] Some student attributes, such as medical knowledge, are readily and effectively assessed by using multiple-choice examinations. Other attributes such as professionalism and clinical and communication skills are best taught and assessed by observing students with patients. Think of a group of young adults who have never played tennis but who want to learn to play well enough to compete in a local tournament. How would you teach them and assess their progress? A lecture followed by a multiple-choice examination seems unlikely to be effective, but instruction while

watching them hitting a tennis ball is much more likely to improve their skills. Recognizing the importance of direct observation, both the Liaison Committee on Medical Education (the body responsible for accrediting medical schools)[2] and the Accreditation Council for Graduate Medical Education (the body responsible for the accreditation of postgraduate medical training)[3] now specifically require assessment that involves direct observation of learners.

Unfortunately, direct observation of students occurs infrequently. A 2004 survey revealed that only 57% of pediatric clerkships evaluate students' physical examinations or other clinical skills by observation.[4] More recently, merely 22% of internal medicine clerkships reported documenting direct observation of students.[5] An in-depth study of a surgery clerkship revealed that faculty evaluated students primarily on the basis of their own interactions with students rather than on observed clinical interactions with patients.[6]

ADVANTAGES OF DIRECT OBSERVATION The aim of direct clinical observation is clear—to help preceptors gather accurate information about students' actual performance in real-life clinical settings rather than inferring performance.[7] Preceptors can then provide effective, timely, and specific feedback on observed skills that can be incorporated into subsequent clinical encounters. With better supervision of learners, both student skills and clinical care improve.[8]

The benefits of increased direct observation are manifold. Students have reported better satisfaction,[9,10] as have preceptors.[11] With faculty development, focusing attention to the process of observation and practice of observation skills, preceptors become more adept at noting specific physical examination and communication skills, and they rate learners' overall performance more consistently.[12] A recent study revealed that as the number of direct observations of medical students in the clerkships increased, preceptor interrater reliability and the correlation between global clinical rating scores, National Board of Medical Examiners subject examination test results, and performance on a fourth-year clinical skills examination all also increased.[13]

OBSERVATION TOOLS Although experienced preceptors may simply observe students in the clinical setting and base feedback on recall, many will use one of the myriad tools designed to help focus observations and direct specific feedback. Observation tools provide a structure that helps faculty focus on skills linked to required learning competencies. In a review of the literature, 55 unique observation tools from 85 studies were described.[14] The majority of tools include items on history taking, physical examination, and communication, although some assess professionalism and behavior. They vary in length from 5 or 6 items to dozens. The tools sometimes use a numerical scale (eg, 1–5) with behavioral anchors for each item. Alternatively, each item may only have a yes/no checkbox (eg, performed or not). Teachers may tailor observation tools for their specific clinical environments.

The tool often used in pediatric education settings is the structured clinical observation (SCO).[11] Although many variations of the SCO exist, most commonly it consists of 3 observation sheets, 1 each for history-taking, information-giving, and physical examination. The history-taking checklist contains 4 domains and 22 items, whereas the physical examination checklist contains only 8 items. Critically, preceptors observing students need only use a single sheet (eg, only history-taking is observed or only physical examination skills are observed). The observation sheets, similar to most observation tools developed for nonevaluative purposes, are designed to allow specific, easy, and quick documentation. The observation score sheets can be completed after 3 to 5 minutes of total observation. The preceptor can then use the score sheets to give focused feedback on an area identified on the scoring sheet that needs remediation.

INCORPORATING OBSERVATION IN CLINICAL PRACTICE The first step to incorporating observation in clinical practice is to create a culture in which observation is understood, expected, nonthreatening, and routine for everyone including patients, parents, students, and preceptors. Preceptors can explain to students during orientation that direct observation is part of the clinical experience.[15] Direct observations should occur regularly, preferably during each clinical session. Frequent short observations are usually better than 1 long observation. Many preceptors find that scheduling medical student observations during the last clinical encounter of the session helps avoid interrupting patient flow. When observing, focus on specific skills and behaviors rather than a global assessment. Observation should target history-taking, communication, and the physical examination skills that match the objectives of the curriculum. For example, all pediatric clerkships expect students to be able to obtain the developmental history of a toddler from a parent but not to counsel about end-of-life issues.

Not all parts of the history or physical examination need to be observed during each clinical encounter. An outpatient preceptor may opt to focus on history-taking and only watch the student obtain the history on the patients seen together in the office that day. An inpatient preceptor may only observe the student obtaining the past medical history, social history, or history of present illness. He or she need not stay for the remainder of the history and physical examination. When using multiple short observations rather than a single long observation, the preceptor commits less time, observes students in a variety of clinical situations, and can monitor how students' skills improve over time. Finally, observation should be coupled with immediate and targeted feedback (the topic of the next Council on Medical Student Education in Pediatrics [COMSEP] Pediatrics Perspectives column) that is based on the observed behaviors.[16]

BARRIERS TO OBSERVATION The 2 most commonly identified barriers are lack of time and training. Although preceptors remain concerned about increased time at work, seeing fewer patients, or lost income,[17] at least 2 recent studies have revealed that direct observation of students does not increase preceptor time.[18,19] Effective observation does require skill. Without appropriate training, preceptors frequently miss errors that students make during observed physical examinations, inconsistently identify students' use of open-ended questions and empathy in medical interviews, and rate students' overall performance inconsistently.[12] The good news is that well-designed faculty development can improve preceptor observation skills.[12]

CONCLUSIONS Focused, direct observation of medical students in clinical settings provides valuable information about learners' skills in history-taking, communication, physical examination, and providing information to children and parents. Observing students' encounters with patients improves teaching, evaluation, preceptor satisfaction, student satisfaction,[20] and, ultimately, patient care. For the great clinical teacher, direct observation is worth the effort.

REFERENCES

1. Council on Medical Student Education in Pediatrics. COMSEP pediatrics clerkship curriculum. Available at: www.comsep.org/Curriculum/pedClerkshipCur.html. Accessed August 20, 2010

2. Liaison Committee on Medical Education. *Functions and Structure of a Medical School: Standards for Accreditation of Medical Education Programs Leading to the MD Degree.* Washington, DC: Association of American Medical Colleges; 2008. Available at: www.lcme.org/functions2008jun.pdf. Accessed August 21, 2010

3. Accreditation Council for Graduate Medical Education. ACGME program requirements for resident education in internal medicine. Available at: www.acgme.org/acWebsite/downloads/RRC_progReq/140_internal_medicine_07012009_TCC.pdf. Accessed August 21, 2010

4. Kumar A, Gera R, Shah G, Godambe S, Kallen DJ. Student evaluation practices in pediatric clerkships: a survey of the medical schools in the United States and Canada. *Clin Pediatr (Phila).* 2004;43(8):729–735

5. Hemmer PA, Papp KK, Mechaber AJ, Durning SJ. Evaluation, grading, and use of the RIME vocabulary on internal medicine clerkships: results of a national survey and comparison to other clinical clerkships. *Teach Learn Med.* 2008;20(2):118–126

6. Pulito AR, Donnelly MB, Plymale M, Mentzer RM Jr. What do faculty observe of medical students' clinical performance? *Teach Learn Med.* 2006;18(2):99–104

7. Worzala K, Rattner SL, Boulet JR, et al. Evaluation of the congruence between students' postencounter notes and standardized patients' checklists in a clinical skills examination. *Teach Learn Med.* 2008; 20(1):31–36

8. Duffy FD, Gordon GH, Whelan G, et al; Participants in the American Academy on Physician and Patient's Conference on Education and Evaluation of Competence in Communication and Interpersonal Skills. Assessing competence in communication and interpersonal skills: the Kalamazoo II report. *Acad Med.* 2004;79(6):495–507

9. Yeung M, Beecker J, Marks M, et al. A new emergency medicine clerkship program: students' perceptions of what works. *CJEM.* 2010;12(3):212–219

10. Kuo AK, Irby DI, Loeser H. Does direct observation improve medical students' clerkship experiences? *Med Educ.* 2005;39(5):518

11. Lane JL, Gottlieb RP. Structured clinical observations: a method to teach clinical skills with limited time and financial resources. *Pediatrics.* 2000;105(4 pt 2):973–977

12. Holmboe ES. Faculty and the observation of trainees' clinical skills: problems and opportunities. *Acad Med.* 2004;79(1):16–22

13. Hasnain M, Connell KJ, Downing SM, Olthoff A, Yudkowsky R. Toward meaningful evaluation of clinical competence: the role of direct observation in clerkship ratings. *Acad Med.* 2004;79(10 suppl):S21–S24

14. Kogan JR, Holmboe ES, Hauer KE. Tools for direct observation and assessment of clinical skills of medical trainees: a systematic review. *JAMA.* 2009;302(12):1316–1326

15. Raszka WV Jr, Maloney CG, Hanson JL. Getting off to a good start: discussing goals and expectations with medical students. *Pediatrics.* 2010;126(2):193–195

16. Fromme HB, Karani R, Downing SM. Direct observation in medical education: a review of the literature and evidence for validity. *Mt Sinai J Med.* 2009;76(4):365–371

17. Levy B, Gjerde C, Albrecht L. The effects of precepting on and the support desired by community-based preceptors in Iowa. *Acad Med.* 1997;72(5):382–384

18. Walters L, Worley P, Prideaux D, Lange K. Do consultations in rural general practice take more time when practitioners are precepting medical students? *Med Educ.* 2008;42(1):69–73

19. Walters L, Prideaux D, Worley P, Greenhill J, Rolfe H. What do general practitioners do differently when consulting with a medical student? *Med Educ.* 2009;43(3):268–273

20. Dolmans DH, Wolfhagen IH, Essed GG, Scherpbier AJ, van der Vleuten CP. The impacts of supervision, patient mix, and numbers of students on the effectiveness of clinical rotations. *Acad Med.* 2002;77(4):332–335

FINANCIAL DISCLOSURE: *The authors have indicated they have no financial relationships relevant to this article to disclose.*

PEDIATRICS PERSPECTIVES

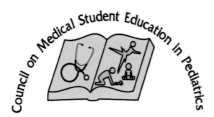

CONTRIBUTORS: Joseph Gigante, MD,[a] Michael Dell, MD,[b] and Angela Sharkey, MD[c]

[a]Department of Pediatrics, Vanderbilt University School of Medicine, Nashville, Tennessee; [b]Department of Pediatrics, Case Western Reserve University School of Medicine, Rainbow Babies & Children's Hospital, Cleveland, Ohio; and [c]Department of Pediatrics, St Louis University School of Medicine, St Louis, Missouri

Address correspondence to Joseph Gigante, MD, Vanderbilt University School of Medicine, 8232 Doctor's Office Tower, Nashville, TN 37232-9225. E-mail: joseph.gigante@vanderbilt.edu

Accepted for publication Nov 19, 2010

doi:10.1542/peds.2010-3351

Getting Beyond "Good Job": How to Give Effective Feedback

This article is the fourth in a series by the Council on Medical Student Education in Pediatrics (COMSEP) reviewing the critical attributes and skills of superb clinical teachers. The previous article in this series reviewed the vital importance of direct observation of students.[1] The purpose of this article is to describe how to use the information gained from the direct observation, namely the role of feedback. Although too often used interchangeably, encouragement, evaluation, and feedback are quite distinct. Encouragement (eg, "good job!") is supportive but does nothing to improve the learner's skills. Evaluation is summative and is the final judgment of the learner's performance. Feedback, however, is designed to improve future performance. This article focuses on feedback—what it is, why it is important, some of the barriers to effective feedback, and how to give helpful feedback.

FEEDBACK: WHAT IT IS

Feedback is an informed, nonevaluative, objective appraisal of performance intended to improve clinical skills.[2] A preceptor can give feedback on history-taking, physical examination, communication, organization, and presentation skills as well as professionalism and written notes.[3] Feedback should provide reassurance about achieved competency, guide future learning, reinforce positive actions, identify and correct areas for improvement, and promote reflection. Effective feedback is specific and describes the observed behavior. Telling a learner that he or she did a good job may reinforce a set of behaviors, but it does not tell the learner which of the observed behaviors should either be repeated or improved. Statements such as "I like how you stated the chief complaint, but the history of present illness needs to include how long the patient has had the complaint and what interventions have made the complaint better or worse" inform the learner of exactly which behavior to repeat, which behavior needs improvement, and how to improve. Feedback concentrates on observed behaviors that can be changed. Telling a learner that he or she is too shy is not useful; however, recommending that the learner be the first to volunteer an answer can be used to change behavior.

Effective feedback is timely, optimally offered immediately after an observed behavior but certainly before the action has been forgotten. If feedback is deferred too long, the learner may forget the context or may not have the opportunity to practice and demonstrate improvement. Effective feedback can be summarized by the acronym STOP (Specific, Timely, Objective and based on Observed behaviors, Plan for improvement discussed with learner).

Three types of feedback exist.[4] Brief feedback occurs daily and is related to an observed action or behavior, such as "let me show you a better way to examine the newborn's abdomen." Formal feedback involves setting aside a specific time for feedback, such as at the end of a presentation on the inpatient service or after a patient encounter in an outpatient clinic. Major feedback occurs during scheduled sessions at strategic points during a clinical rotation, usually at the midpoint, and serves to provide more comprehensive information to the learner so that he or she can improve before the end of the rotation, when the final evaluation is performed.

FEEDBACK: WHY IT IS IMPORTANT

The ability to give feedback effectively is one of the defining characteristics of master teachers.[5] In the absence of feedback from experienced preceptors, learners are left to rely on self-assessment to determine what has gone well and what needs improvement. Although effective feedback promotes self-assessment, studies have shown that inexperienced learners do not consistently identify their own strengths and weaknesses.[2,6] Learners may also interpret an absence of feedback as implicit approval of their performance. Simply put, without appropriate feedback, clinical skills cannot improve. Because medical training uses a system of gradually diminishing supervision, uncorrected mistakes early in training may be perpetuated and even taught to subsequent learners. Timely feedback, therefore, has important implications not only for learning but also for high-quality patient care.

BARRIERS TO FEEDBACK

Despite its critical role in professional development, learners regularly report receiving little feedback on their performance.[7] Many barriers to providing effective feedback have been reported.[7,8] Clinical preceptors may not be involved in curriculum development, so they may be uncomfortable defining expectations for their learners.[9] Brief encounters with learners and busy patient schedules may offer limited opportunity for direct observation of learners.[1] Preceptors may have incomplete or inaccurate concepts of what constitutes feedback. Learners, for their part, may not recognize feedback when it is offered. Finally, many people find it easier to offer positive encouragement instead of constructive feedback, a tendency only reinforced when the latter is met with defensiveness from learners. Another major barrier is perceived lack of time.[6,10] Depending on the situation, formal or major feedback may take 5 to 20 minutes. However, brief focused feedback takes little time and is highly effective.[4]

FEEDBACK: HOW TO DO IT WELL

There are a number of techniques for providing feedback to learners.[2,4,8,11,12] A frequently used method is the "feedback sandwich." The top slice of bread is a positive comment (ie, about what the learner has done well); the middle of the sandwich is an area of improvement (ie, what the learner needs to improve); and the bottom slice of bread is another positive comment, which ends the session on an upbeat note. Although this format is often used, other techniques promote self-reflection and may be more effective and engaging,[6,13] which is particularly true for learners with poor performance.[14]

On the basis of experience gained from Council on Medical Student Education in Pediatrics workshops and a review of the current literature, we recommend the following 5-step framework for giving formal and major feedback (Table 1).

1. Outline the expectations for the learner during orientation.[9] Learners cannot succeed if they do not know what is expected of them.

2. Prepare the learner to receive feedback. Learners often state that they receive little feedback,[7] whereas

TABLE 1 Guidelines for Giving Feedback

Outline the expectations for the learner
Prepare the learner to receive feedback
  Use the word "feedback"
  Make feedback private
  Make feedback timely
Ask the learner for self-assessment
  Make feedback interactive
Tell the learner how he or she is doing
  Base feedback on observed actions and
    changeable behaviors
  Provide concrete examples
Agree on a plan for improvement
  Allow learner to react to feedback
  Suggest specific ways to improve performance
  Develop an action plan with learner; elicit
    suggestions from learner
  Outline consequences

educators report consistently giving feedback.[15] Bridge this gap with the phrase, "I am giving you feedback." Specifically using the word "feedback" helps the learner recognize the intent.[4] To minimize discomfort or embarrassment and promote a dialogue, feedback should be given in a private setting.

3. Ask learners how they think they are performing. Encouraging learners to assess and correct their own performance routinely helps them to develop the skills of lifelong learning and leads to a shared view of what needs improvement.[13]

4. Tell the learner how you think he or she is doing. Feedback should be based on specific, observed actions and changeable behaviors. Provide concrete examples of what the learner did well and what the learner could improve. The feedback needs to be appropriate to the curriculum and the developmental stage of the learner.

5. Develop a plan for improvement. The learner should have the opportunity to comment on the feedback and make his or her own suggestions for improvement. The preceptor can then suggest additional

ways to improve learner performance. The learner and preceptor can then develop an action plan for improvement together.

Ideally, brief feedback should occur daily. For preceptors, remembering to "STOP" for a moment to give feedback may enhance the frequency and effectiveness of feedback. Faculty-development programs can help preceptors understand expectations for students and overcome anxiety about giving feedback.[16] Course or program directors can e-mail or notify preceptors of the need to give major feedback at the midpoint of the rotation. Preceptors may designate a day of the week for feedback (eg, Feedback Fridays).[11] Finally, learners themselves can be encouraged to take the initiative to elicit feedback by either asking for it verbally or asking their preceptor to fill out a form or a clinical encounter card.[17]

CONCLUSIONS
Effective feedback is critical for improving the clinical performance of medical students and residents. It provides learners with information on past performances so that future performance can be improved. Ulti-

mately, not only does effective feedback help our learners but our patients as well. Feedback is a critical skill for educators that is necessary and valuable and, after some practice and planning, can be incorporated into daily practice.[2]

ACKNOWLEDGMENTS
We thank our editors Susan Bannister and William Raszka for their helpful comments and thoughtful reviews of the manuscript.

REFERENCES
1. Hanson JL, Bannister SL, Clark A, Raszka WV Jr. Oh, what you can see: the role of observation in medical student education. Pediatrics. 2010;126(5):843–845
2. Ende J. Feedback in clinical medical education. JAMA. 1983;250(6):777–781
3. Spickard A, 3rd, Gigante J, Stein G, Denny JC. Automatic capture of student notes to augment mentor feedback and student performance on patient write-ups. J Gen Intern Med. 2008;23(7):979–984
4. Branch WTJ, Paranjape A. Feedback and reflection: teaching methods for clinical settings. Acad Med. 2002;77(12 pt 1):1185–1188
5. Torre DM, Simpson D, Sebastian JL, Elnicki DM. Learning/feedback activities and high-quality teaching: perceptions of third-year medical students during an inpatient rotation. Acad Med. 2005;80(10):950–954
6. Sachdeva AK. Use of effective feedback to facilitate adult learning. J Cancer Educ. 1996;11(2):106–118
7. Gil DH, Heins M, Jones PB. Perceptions of

medical school faculty members and students on clinical clerkship feedback. J Med Educ. 1984;59(11 pt 1):856–864
8. Irby DM. What clinical teachers in medicine need to know. Acad Med. 1994;69(5):333–342
9. Raszka WV Jr, Maloney CG, Hanson JL. Getting off to a good start: discussing goals and expectations with medical students. Pediatrics. 2010;126(2):193–195
10. Schurn T, Yindra K. Relationship between systematic feedback to faculty and ratings of clinical teaching. Acad Med. 1996;71(10):1100–1102
11. Bing-You RG, Bertsch T, Thompson JA. Coaching medical students in receiving effective feedback. Teach Learn Med. 1997;10(4):228–231
12. Hewson MG, Little ML. Giving feedback in medical education: verification of recommended techniques. J Gen Intern Med. 1998;13(2):111–116
13. Cantillon P, Sargeant J. Giving feedback in clinical settings. BMJ. 2008;337:a1961
14. Milan FB, Parish SJ, Reichgott MJ. A model for educational feedback based on clinical communication skills strategies: beyond the "feedback sandwich." Teach Learn Med. 2006;18(1):42–47
15. Gibson C. Promoting effective teaching and learning: hospital consultants identify their needs. Med Educ. 2000;34(2):126–130
16. Brukner H, Altkorn D, Cook S, Quinn M, McNabb W. Giving effective feedback to medical students: a workshop for faculty and housestaff. Med Teach. 1999;21(2):161–165
17. Greenberg LW. Medical students' perceptions of feedback in a busy ambulatory setting: a descriptive study using a clinical encounter card. South Med J. 2004;97(12):1174–1178

FINANCIAL DISCLOSURE: The authors have indicated they have no financial relationships relevant to this article to disclose.

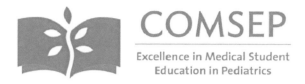

AUTHORS: Stacey Bernstein, MD, FRCPC,[a,b] Adelle R. Atkinson, MD, FRCPC,[a,b] and Maria Athina Martimianakis, PhD[a,b]

[a]Hospital for Sick Children, Toronto, Ontario, Canada; and [b]Department of Pediatrics, University of Toronto, Toronto, Ontario, Canada

Address correspondence to Stacey Bernstein, MD, FRCPC, Department of Pediatrics, Hospital for Sick Children, 555 University Ave, Toronto, ON, Canada M5G 1X8. E-mail: stacey.bernstein@sickkids.ca

Accepted for publication May 17, 2013

doi:10.1542/peds.2013-1526

Diagnosing the Learner in Difficulty

Teaching undergraduate and postgraduate learners is often a joy. What to do with a student who is not meeting expectations, however, is challenging. Clinical attending physicians must identify, and remediate, students who struggle. This article presents a practical approach to identifying, diagnosing, and managing the learner in difficulty.

DEFINING AT-RISK STUDENTS

A learner in difficulty is a student at risk for receiving less than "pass" because of concerns regarding his or her knowledge base, clinical skills, or professionalism.[1] Learners in difficulty rarely self-identify for a variety of reasons, including lack of self-awareness or concern that if they acknowledge they are in difficulty, they will be stigmatized.[2] However, early identification of such individuals, with appropriate intervention, seems to lead to better outcomes for these learners.[3] The responsibility of identifying learners who are not meeting expectations largely rests with their clinical teachers.

THE CHALLENGE FOR CLINICAL TEACHERS

Many teachers hesitate to identify and report learners experiencing difficulties for a number of reasons, including inexperience handling such situations, concern they are misjudging the circumstances, lack of documentation, fear of retribution by the student, and

the time required to resolve issues.[4–6] The current nature of training further compounds this problem. Oversaturated placements, shorter duty hours and academic half days, and concurrent exposure to multiple supervisors reduce student contact with clinical teachers. Problems often go unidentified until a critical incident has occurred.[6]

THE APPROACH

Just as we all have an approach to a child who presents with a cough, it is helpful to have a basic approach to a learner who is not meeting expectations. Teachers are good at recognizing a student not doing well but have difficulty deciding what to do next. We propose that the steps should be analogous to those of a physician confronted with a coughing patient: consider a differential diagnosis, take a focused history, observe, and define a management plan.

CASE

Julie is a fourth-year medical student working as an acting intern. The supervising resident reports that Julie seems distracted and disorganized, and has a weak knowledge base. The clinical attending has noticed that she appears distracted and disinterested but has not appreciated any knowledge deficits. Julie's interactions with

other members of the health care team have been acceptable.

Recognizing that Julie is not meeting the expectations, the clinical attending needs to develop a differential diagnosis for why Julie is struggling (Table 1). Taking a careful history of a learner such as Julie and gathering focused observations will narrow the differential and help the attending decide on a working diagnosis and therapeutic plan.

CONSTRUCTING A DIFFERENTIAL

The reasons why learners struggle are diverse and are often not academic in origin.[7] Moreover, unlike a clinical differential, in which there is usually 1 explanation for the patient's presentation, the struggling learner may be dealing with several issues. Learning is relational; thus, to determine what may be causing problems for a learner such as Julie, it is important to consider what, if any, interactions a student may be having in the learning context that could be interfering with his or her performance. When constructing a differential diagnosis of a learner in difficulty, the acronym "K-Salts" (knowledge, skills, attitude, learner, teacher, system)[2] is useful. This approach allows the attending to think not only of the skills, attitudes, and behaviors of the learner but also to consider the impact of the environment.

TABLE 1 A Differential Diagnosis of the Learner Not Meeting Expectations

Factors	Topics to Consider	Examples From the Case
Knowledge	Deficiencies in the basic and/or clinical sciences; anxiety; sleep deprivation	Below-expectations knowledge base (as per resident)
Skills	Difficulty interpreting information, clinical reasoning and organization; poor relationships with patients	Is disorganized
Attitude	Lack of motivation or insight	Distracted and disinterested
Learner	Stress, learning disability, substance abuse, mental illness	Stressed over performance and personal issues
Teacher	Teacher may be dissatisfied with his or her own role, may be experiencing own stresses or biases	Has not observed student very much
System	Overwhelming workload, inconsistency of teaching/supervision, reduced clinical exposure	No systems issues seem to be impacting student's learning

TAKING THE HISTORY

When talking to a student who is not meeting expectations, start with open-ended questions to determine his or her level of insight into problems and potential causal factors. As the conversation progresses, some key areas to explore include:

1. Academic history: to determine how well the student is handling the academic requirements of training (eg, study habits, competing priorities such as research projects, call requirements).

2. Social circumstances: to determine if any recent or ongoing life stressors are interfering with learning (eg, financial, child care issues, illnesses in the immediate or extended family).

3. Wellness: to determine if there are any new or previously known physical and/or mental health issues that are contributing to the concerns identified.

4. Academic relationships: to determine if relationships with other students or attitudes of teachers may be impeding success.

5. Learning context: to identify if any organizational or systems issues are interfering with learning (eg, inconsistent supervision, poor role modeling, overcrowded learning environments, geographically dispersed teaching sites).

A CONVERSATION WITH JULIE MIGHT REVEAL THE FOLLOWING:

Julie is married and has a 2-year-old son who attends day care near her home. Her husband works full-time. She has a 1-hour commute to work and finds it hard to be there on time to pick up her son from day care. Furthermore, her son has been ill, requiring her husband to miss work, and she has been up late at night. She is having difficulty balancing her personal and professional responsibilities and is stressed that she is not doing a good job either at home or at work. Julie feels rushed and tired, and she finds it hard to organize her day. She has never experienced this before and is embarrassed that the team has noticed.

OBSERVING THE STUDENT

Although the history is critically important to understanding Julie's issues, observation enables the attending to better understand the learner's performance.

Observing Julie admitting an infant with failure to thrive might reveal the following: Julie has a good rapport with the mother but takes a scattered history. She writes her admission note before entering any admission orders,

resulting in a delay. Her presentation during rounds is not well organized, and her differential diagnosis for the failure to thrive is rudimentary.

MAKING THE DIAGNOSIS

Julie is having difficulty balancing her home and professional life; in addition, she has problems with organization and prioritization, and has knowledge deficits. Although Julie's problems are multifactorial, the clinical attending now has a much better understanding of the issues and can offer specific suggestions for improvement.

MANAGEMENT

In addition to offering specific advice, the clinical attending has 2 other critical responsibilities. First, the teacher must document the concerns and what has been done about them, in as much detail as possible (ie, dates, specific circumstances, conversations with other members of the health care team). Second, the clinical teacher should notify a responsible authority in the medical student or residency program. In this way, the teacher can learn if this is an isolated incident or a trend, and greater resources for intervention may be available.

HELPFUL TIPS

- If the learner identifies personal health issues as a contributing factor, guide him or her to the Student Affairs or Wellness office.

- Ask for help. The clerkship director, residency program director, education site leader, or associate dean will want to assist you and the learner.

- Know your school's regulations and guidelines about struggling or failing students. Know whom to contact. Know the supports that are available to both you and your students.

You discuss Julie's situation, and she highlights the multiple issues involved. You suggest that Julie seek advice from the Student Affairs office, and she agrees that this is a good plan. You also suggest some resources to increase her pediatric knowledge. Together, you agree that you will speak to the pediatric Clerkship Director to convey your concerns about the impact of her long commute on her learning. Julie wonders if she could be transferred to the community hospital that is closer to her home; you agree that this would be a good plan.

CONCLUSIONS

As clinical teachers, we have an obligation to both our profession and society to identify, and assist, students who struggle to meet the standards expected of them. The good news is that close to 90% of students labeled as "learners in difficulty" succeed after implementation of a structured intervention, especially if they are involved in developing the remediation plan.[8]

ACKNOWLEDGMENTS

The authors thank Drs Susan Bannister, Robert Dudas, and Christopher Maloney for their thoughtful critique and editing of the manuscript.

REFERENCES

1. Frellsen SL, Baker EA, Papp KK, Durning SJ. Medical school policies regarding struggling medical students during the internal medicine clerkships: results of a national survey. *Acad Med.* 2008;83(9):876–881

2. Steinert Y. The "problem" learner: whose problem is it? AMEE guide no. 76. *Med Teach.* 2013;35(4):e1035–e1045

3. Yao DC, Wright SM. The challenge of problem residents. *J Gen Intern Med.* 2001;16(7):486–492

4. Dudek NL, Marks MB, Regehr G. Failure to fail: the perspectives of clinical supervisors. *Acad Med.* 2005;80(suppl 10):S84–S87

5. McGraw R, Verma S. The trainee in difficulty. *CJEM.* 2001;3(3):205–208

6. Evans DE, Alstead EM, Brown J. Applying your clinical skills to students and trainees in academic difficulty. *Clin Teach.* 2010;7(4):230–235

7. Sayer M, Chaput De Saintonge M, Evans D, Wood D. Support for students with academic difficulties. *Med Educ.* 2002;36(7):643–650

8. Reamy BV, Harman JH. Residents in trouble: an in-depth assessment of the 25-year experience of a single family medicine residency. *Fam Med.* 2006;38(4):252–257

FINANCIAL DISCLOSURE: *The authors have indicated they have no financial relationships relevant to this article to disclose.*
FUNDING: No external funding.

Assessment for Learning: How to Assess Your Learners' Performance in the Clinical Environment

Janice L. Hanson, PhD, EdS, MH,[b,c] Colleen M. Wallace, MD,[a] Susan L. Bannister, MD, Med[d]

"Learner assessment" usually refers to assigning ratings and writing comments on forms at the end of a rotation. Although these are important aspects of assessment, assessment can begin the moment a preceptor meets a learner, and it can set the stage for a meaningful learning experience. Whether the time together is one half-day session or several weeks, preceptors who assess their learners' competence, knowledge, and interests "in the moment" can help target their teaching to the learners' goals and needs. This article, which is next in the series by the Council on Medical Student Education in Pediatrics about the skills of great clinical teachers, provides strategies for an "Assessment for Learning."

ASSESSMENT FOR LEARNING: WHAT IS IT?

Assessment encompasses gathering data about a learner's performance through observation and interactions, providing feedback, recording observations and ratings, and synthesizing data to make summary recommendations about a learner. Assessment for learning, sometimes called formative assessment, includes those aspects of assessment that shape the learner's abilities.[1] Clinical teachers are ideally suited to assess for learning in clinical work environments, beginning in the first moments when meeting a learner.[2]

The benefits of assessing a learner's knowledge, abilities, and goals at the beginning of a teaching interaction include the following:

1. Preceptors are better able to teach to the learner's level and help them progress.

2. Preceptors are better equipped to help the learner address individual learning goals.

3. Preceptors can help prepare an "educational sign out" or "teaching handover" that they, or the learner, give to the next preceptor to allow both the teacher to be prepared and the learner to continue their learning trajectory.[3]

4. Preceptors are better able to write high-quality, helpful narrative comments, facilitating future learner progress and assisting clerkship directors and grading committees in monitoring learners' progress.[4] When making some quick observations and assessments in the moment, a preceptor can use them in real time to teach but then also scribble a quick note. Then, when it comes time to complete an evaluation form, the preceptor can use the notes to provide specific examples in comments for summative assessment.

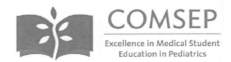

[a]Departments of Pediatrics and [b]Medicine, Office of Education, Washington University in Saint Louis, Saint Louis, Missouri; [c]Departments of Medicine and Pediatrics, Uniformed Services University of the Health Sciences, Bethesda, Maryland; [d]Department of Pediatrics, University of Calgary, Calgary, Alberta, Canada

Drs Hanson and Bannister conceptualized the article and drafted the initial manuscript; Dr Wallace contributed important concepts to the article and edited the initial manuscript; and all authors reviewed and revised the manuscript, and approved the final manuscript as submitted, and agree to be accountable for all aspects of the work.

DOI: https://doi.org/10.1542/peds.2019-3966

Accepted for publication Dec 16, 2019

Address correspondence to Janice L. Hanson, PhD, EdS, MH, Washington University in Saint Louis, Room 320, Becker Library, Campus Box 8214, 660 S Euclid Ave, Saint Louis, MO 63110. E-mail: janicehanson@wustl.edu

PEDIATRICS (ISSN Numbers: Print, 0031-4005; Online, 1098-4275).

FINANCIAL DISCLOSURE: The authors have indicated they have no financial relationships relevant to this article to disclose.

FUNDING: No external funding.

POTENTIAL CONFLICT OF INTEREST: The authors have indicated they have no potential conflicts of interest to disclose.

To cite: Hanson JL, Wallace CM, Bannister SL. Assessment for Learning: How to Assess Your Learners' Performance in the Clinical Environment. *Pediatrics.* 2020;145(3):e20193966

STRATEGIES FOR ASSESSMENT FOR LEARNING

Elicit Goals

Course objectives and evaluation forms are a great place to begin the conversation about learning goals because they provide a framework and clear outline of expectations. Preceptors and trainees can devise a plan of which topics to focus on during the clinical experience. Inquiring about personal interests, career goals, and learning goals (eg, specific physical examination techniques, presentation skills, or clinical reasoning) can also help guide and individualize teaching while providing insight into the learner's approach to self-assessment.

Use Direct Observation

Although it may not be realistic to observe learners doing all their clinical work, observations can focus on parts of the history, specific physical examination skills, interacting with patients, sharing information with families, or coordinating with team members. Observations of even a few minutes will add insight about current performance and appropriate next steps.[5,6]

Assess While You Teach

While caring for patients together, preceptors can focus the learner on specific patient care goals by asking, "What is the most important thing we need to know about this patient to help us determine the best management plan?" (For some patients, it is the presence or absence of fever, results of blood tests, evolution of a rash, or need for oxygen.) The student's reply can assist the preceptor in determining how the learner is approaching clinical reasoning for this patient.[7] The preceptor can then adjust the conversation to the knowledge level of the trainee.

Another approach is "Learn Something New Every Day" rounds. All team members (students, residents, nurses, and preceptors) take turns sharing something they learned recently. For a large team, set a time limit of 60 seconds for each person's "teaching pearl" to keep the discussion short. This strategy allows each team member to practice teaching and also provides an authentic opportunity to model and practice lifelong learning. In addition, this approach gives preceptors an opportunity to assess learners' knowledge, communication skills, and motivation.

Reviewing clinical guidelines or protocols provides another method to both assess and teach in an outpatient clinic, hospital unit, or newborn nursery by encouraging learners to think aloud about why pediatricians do what they do. For example, in the newborn nursery, education about hypoglycemia guidelines can begin with asking learners questions such as, "Which infants are at risk for low blood glucose?"; "Why?"; "What is the pathophysiology?"; "How long would that risk last?" For hyperbilirubinemia guidelines, ask, "Which infants are at risk for jaundice?"; "When or how often do we measure their bilirubin?"; "At what point do we start phototherapy?" This strategy helps preceptors assess learners' understanding of disease process, epidemiology, and rationale for evaluation and management and then guide teaching to the appropriate level for each topic.

Activities as straightforward as discussing a clinical case or an approach to a chief complaint ("2 month old with wheezing" or "15 year old with abdominal pain") can also provide an opportunity to assess the learner's knowledge and clinical reasoning while discussing the differential diagnosis, evaluation,

TABLE 1 Assessment for Learning

Elicit goals
  Question to elicit goals
    What aspects of pediatrics relate to your career goals and interests?
    What knowledge or skill do you hope to focus on during your time in this clinic (or working with this team)?
Use direct observation
  Spend several minutes watching the learner care for a patient while assessing a particular skill
    History taking (eg, past medical history, family history, or social history)
    A physical examination technique (eg, respiratory, abdominal, or ear)
    Information sharing (eg, anticipatory guidance or instructions for medications)
    Communication skills with patients and families
    Coordination of care with team members
Assess while you teach
  Ask, "What is the most important thing we need to know about this patient to help us determine the best management plan?"
  Use Learn Something New Every Day rounds, in which everyone on the team shares something they have learned recently (in ≤60 s)
  Think aloud about clinical guidelines or protocols
  Assess clinical reasoning while talking through the differential diagnosis, evaluation, and management plan (about actual patients or hypothetical patients)
Compare the learner's performance to a framework
  Summarize observations with the RIME framework: How does this learner primarily function?
    Reporter (gathers and presents patient data)
    Interpreter (interprets and prioritizes patient data)
    Manager (creates a plan for patient care)
    Educator (educates self, patients, and team members)
Look to the future
  Help a learner set new learning goals
  Create a teaching handover with the learner (plans for learning and requesting feedback in the next clinical experience)
  Share assessment for learning observations in comments on evaluation forms

and management plan. Learners can ask clarifying questions about the patient, and the teacher and learner can discuss the clinical reasoning of why different diagnoses may be higher or lower on the list depending on the answers.[8]

Compare the Learner's Performance to a Framework

The reporter, interpreter, manager, educator (RIME) framework provides a practical way to synthesize an assessment while working with a student.[4,8] The RIME framework helps clinical teachers look for patterns in each learner's competence in clinical care. A reliable reporter consistently and accurately gathers the data needed for patient care and presents it in a clear and organized way. An interpreter interprets what the information means for patient diagnosis and care. A manager consistently proposes, discusses, and implements treatment plans. An educator educates himself or herself, patients, or others about each patient's diagnosis and care needs. The RIME framework helps preceptors summarize their observations about the learner's abilities, identify the level in the framework at which the learner generally performs, and outline a plan for improvement.

Look to the Future

Preceptors who have engaged in assessment for learning are well positioned to help learners create specific goals regarding physical examination or communication skills, interpretation of laboratory results, knowledge of clinical guidelines and how to apply them, or other aspects of clinical reasoning and care that have been observed, taught, and discussed. Preceptors can assist learners in self-assessing their own learning, articulating refined goals for their next clinical experience, defining specific feedback they can request from another teacher, and determining how they will decide whether they have succeeded in meeting their goals.

CONCLUSIONS

Assessment for learning, developed and practiced in observations and teaching in the clinical setting, forms a strong foundation for shaping a learner's progress (Table 1). The same observations and guidance for learning form the basis for high-quality comments on evaluation forms, whether the teacher and learner spend a few hours or a few weeks working together. Specific examples of what the learner said and did while caring for patients benefit everyone: the teacher who assesses and guides, the learner who progresses and forms new goals, and the program leader who makes decisions about the learner's readiness for the next steps along the path of education.

ABBREVIATION

RIME: reporter, interpreter, manager, educator

REFERENCES

1. Pangaro LN, McGaghie WC, eds. *Handbook on Medical Student Evaluation and Assessment.* North Syracuse, NY: Gegensatz Press; 2015

2. Norcini J, Burch V. Workplace-based assessment as an educational tool: AMEE Guide No. 31. *Med Teach.* 2007; 29(9):855–871

3. Fuchs J, King M, Devon EP, Guffey D, Keeley M, Rocha MEM. Mitigating "Educational Groundhog Day" - the role of learner handoffs within clinical rotations: a survey of pediatric educational leaders [published online ahead of print August 22, 2019]. *Acad Pediatr.* doi:10.1016/j.acap.2019.08.011

4. Holmes AV, Peltier CB, Hanson JL, Lopreiato JO. Writing medical student and resident performance evaluations: beyond "performed as expected". *Pediatrics.* 2014;133(5):766–768

5. Lane JL, Gottlieb RP. Structured clinical observations: a method to teach clinical skills with limited time and financial resources. *Pediatrics.* 2000;105(4, pt 2): 973–977

6. Hanson JL, Bannister SL, Clark A, Raszka WV Jr.. Oh, what you can see: the role of observation in medical student education. *Pediatrics.* 2010;126(5): 843–845

7. Stuart E, Hanson JL, Dudas RA. The right stuff: priming students to focus on pertinent information during clinical encounters. *Pediatrics.* 2019;144(1): e20191311

8. Dell M, Lewin L, Gigante J. What's the story? Expectations for oral case presentations. *Pediatrics.* 2012;130(1): 1–4

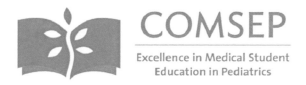

AUTHORS: Alison Volpe Holmes, MD, MPH,[a,b] Christopher B. Peltier, MD,[c,d] Janice L. Hanson, PhD,[e] and Joseph O. Lopreiato, MD, MPH[f]

[a]The Children's Hospital at Dartmouth, Lebanon, New Hampshire; [b]Department of Pediatrics, the Geisel School of Medicine at Dartmouth, Hanover, New Hampshire; [c]Cincinnati Children's Hospital Medical Center; [d]Department of Pediatrics, University of Cincinnati College of Medicine, Cincinnati, Ohio; [e]Department of Pediatrics, University of Colorado School of Medicine, Denver, Colorado; and [f]Department of Pediatrics, Uniformed Services University of the Health Sciences, Bethesda, Maryland

Address correspondence to Alison V. Holmes, MD, MPH, Dartmouth-Hitchcock Medical Center, Pediatrics, Rubin 552, One Medical Center Dr, Lebanon, NH 03756. E-mail: Alison.V.Holmes@hitchcock.org

Accepted for publication Feb 13, 2014

KEY WORDS
competency-based education; students, medical; education, medical, undergraduate

ABBREVIATIONS
PRIME+—professionalism, reporter, interpreter, manager, educator, plus suggesting an area for focused improvement and development.
RIME—reporter, interpreter, manager, educator

Dr Holmes wrote the original first draft of the article; did most of the re-drafting of the article; sought, read, and reviewed all the references; and led the process of rewrites with the Council on Medical Student Education in Pediatrics editorial committee; Drs Peltier and Lopreiato contributed much of the content to the outline of the first draft of the article, assisted with multiple re-drafts of the article, and wrote individual sections of the article; Dr Hanson contributed substantial new content to the article, assisted with multiple re-drafts of the article, and wrote individual sections of the article; and all authors approved the final manuscript as submitted.

doi:10.1542/peds.2014-0418

Writing Medical Student and Resident Performance Evaluations: Beyond "Performed as Expected"

This article continues the Council on Medical Student Education in Pediatrics' series on the skills of, and strategies used by, excellent clinical teachers. Here, we provide a practical framework and helpful tips for writing student evaluations that will inform both students and their medical schools.

—Susan Bannister, Editor, Council on Medical Student Education in Pediatrics Monthly Feature

In the present age of competency-based evaluations, faculty complete more forced-choice performance rating scales. Nonetheless, the narrative evaluation that tells the "story" of the learner remains critical, providing context that helps students understand the

feedback they receive and clerkship directors understand the "big picture" of each student's performance. For medical students, narrative evaluations can be included in the Medical Student Performance Evaluation that summarizes their performance in the first 3 years of medical school and becomes part of their residency applications. In this article, we review a framework that can help preceptors write narratives that more fully reflect observed performance.

THE CURRENT STATE OF EVALUATIONS: DIFFICULT TO INTERPRET

Despite many clinical observations, intelligent and accomplished faculty

can suffer writer's block when trying to write meaningful descriptions of students.[1] Consider the following examples that we have received:

> "Needs to work on follow-through of plans and communicating with staff. Will refer to clerkship director."

> "Very pleasant. Fun to work with. Seemed to enjoy Ped ED setting. Overall, performed as expected."

> "Exceeded all expectations. Very bright and organized."

> "Although a likable person, at times he appeared to be confused during the rotation."

> "Development of treatment plans will improve with experience. Continue reading to improve fund of knowledge"

Although truthful and honest, these written narratives do not provide enough information on current performance and do not specify areas for focused attention in subsequent learning experiences.

A TOOL TO HELP WRITE BETTER STUDENT EVALUATIONS

A widely used tool for improving written evaluations was developed by Dr Louis Pangaro at the Uniformed Services University. Known as RIME, it classifies important observable trainee behaviors and skills into 4 easily observed domains: reporter, interpreter, manager, and educator.[2] In an individual clinical encounter, learners may demonstrate behaviors from several domains.[3]

THE RIME FRAMEWORK: A REVIEW

"R" for reporter refers to the student's ability to obtain information from a patient or family interview, to review a medical record, and to report findings coherently in oral presentations and written notes.

Interpreter is the "I" in RIME. This domain addresses how well a learner can interpret data collected from the history, physical examination, medical record, laboratory data, and radiologic studies; prioritize the most urgent problems; and formulate a well-reasoned differential diagnosis.

RIME continues with "M" for manager. As a manager, a student would formulate diagnostic and therapeutic patient plans and manage all aspects of care for the most common complaints. Management includes performing simple procedures and managing one's own time.

The "E" in RIME is for educator, which includes students' abilities to educate themselves via self-directed learning, appropriately accepting and responding to feedback, and critical interpretation of the medical literature. Students can teach by locating relevant articles, and also can teach patients about health conditions.

RIME AND PRIME+

As Pangaro described reporter, interpreter, manager, and educator, professionalism was explicitly incorporated within each domain.[4] We propose the addition of a "P" to RIME to specifically highlight professionalism; with this reminder, professionalism is less apt to be omitted from written narratives. The "P" reminds evaluators to incorporate comments about professionalism into each RIME domain. A "plus" at the end reminds the evaluator to suggest an area for focused improvement and development, giving students feedback that will help them progress along the continuum of medical education.[3,5,6]

USING THE LANGUAGE OF PRIME+ IN WRITTEN NARRATIVES

Here are 2 good examples of narrative comments that use the PRIME+ framework to provide useful descriptions of students' performance. With several descriptions like this, a clerkship director could assess a student's progress, provide meaningful feedback to the student about performance in the clerkship, and formulate strong statements for the Medical Student Performance Evaluation.

Jane was always on time, reliable, and dependable such that I always knew the information she provided was accurate. She was able to report data succinctly and gather complete histories while simultaneously maintaining excellent rapport with families. She performed good differential diagnoses, was able to interpret lab data, PFTs, etc, and to independently find resources to help her when she came across data she had not encountered previously. Jane could synthesize good plans, and managed patients well, always spending additional time to ensure family understanding of instructions. She responded well to feedback with appreciation and an upbeat attitude, worked diligently on fund of knowledge, and was able to educate families and patients well on various illnesses; always the professional, spending more time and effort whenever it was required by the situation.

Professionally, John was prompt, appropriately groomed, friendly, and had an energetic style much appreciated by patients and staff. As a reporter, John needs to continue to work on completeness and organization; excellent efforts are made, but he can lose the big picture by focusing on the wrong detail. As an interpreter, he continues to have short differentials and elementary understanding of how to organize and evaluate complex, or multiproblem patients. Manager skills are adequate, as John generally did well calling back patients and following up on labs and studies, and did not fall behind on documentation. He needs to continue to develop longer-term planning for more complex patients; having trouble synthesizing different aspects of psychosocial dimensions all pertaining to 1 patient. Educator: John reviewed a randomized trial on 2 different steroids in the treatment of asthma. He seemed minimally prepared and had only very basic understanding of how to interpret and use information from an RCT. Of many potential areas of improvement, would start in the reporter domain by increasing details in histories, increasing completeness of histories, and overall organization of presentations.

USING PRIME+ IN DAILY PRACTICE

Once familiar with PRIME+, a busy pediatrician can keep short daily notes on learners in each of the domains. Office-based preceptors, who often work one-on-one with students, can use these notes to give formative feedback after each encounter or at the end of the day. Hospital-based pediatricians can keep a PRIME+ table of learners on their team, and then use these organized notes to write evaluations. Because RIME domains relate directly to the work of a physician, the framework helps a preceptor organize observations from daily work into a useful narrative. When listening on rounds or reading notes, teachers can assess reporter skills. In taking an overnight phone call from a student, one can note interpretation of patient data. Manager skills can be evaluated via timely completion of office visits or in coordination of patient care. In all interactions, the teacher can be actively considering where the student is in relation to curriculum goals, and what he or she needs to do to progress to the next level.

CONCLUSIONS

Written narratives can be challenging to write and are critically important in medical student and resident education. PRIME+ can provide structure for observation, formative feedback, and for writing summative evaluations at the end of a clinical experience. Using PRIME+ to structure your observations and evaluations, written narratives can be more effective, specific, and meaningful.

REFERENCES

1. Lye PS, Biernat KA, Bragg DS, Simpson DE. A pleasure to work with—an analysis of written comments on student evaluations. *Ambul Pediatr.* 2001;1(3):128–131

2. Pangaro L. A new vocabulary and other innovations for improving descriptive in-training evaluations. *Acad Med.* 1999;74(11):1203–1207

3. Pangaro L, Holmboe ES. *Evaluation Forms and Global Rating Scales. Practical Guide to the Evaluation of Clinical Competence.* Philadelphia, PA: Mosby Elsevier; 2008:24–41

4. Pangaro LN. A shared professional framework for anatomy and clinical clerkships. *Clin Anat.* 2006;19(5):419–428

5. Hicks PJ, Schumacher DJ, Benson BJ, et al. The pediatrics milestones: conceptual framework, guiding principles, and approach to development. *J Grad Med Educ.* 2010;2(3):410–418

6. The Association of American Medical Colleges. AAMC Pediatric program focuses on competency-based learning. Available at: https://www.aamc.org/newsroom/newsreleases/343836/05312013.html#.UrhA3yize2w. Accessed December 23, 2013

FINANCIAL DISCLOSURE: The authors have indicated they have no financial relationships relevant to this article to disclose.
FUNDING: No external funding.
POTENTIAL CONFLICT OF INTEREST: The authors have indicated they have no potential conflicts of interest to disclose.

The LETTER of Recommendation: Showcasing a Student's Strengths

Erin Pete Devon, MD,[a] Rebekah Burns, MD,[b] Amanda Hartke, MD, PhD[c,d]

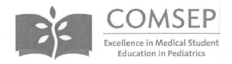

As you wrap up your end-of-rotation feedback with a student, the student asks hesitantly, "Would you be willing to write me a strong recommendation letter for residency?" Your internal monologue starts to alarm: "Should I say yes? What makes a strong letter? I've never done this before! Where do I even start?" This article, next in the Council on Medical Student Education in Pediatrics series on teaching medical students, will help you approach this important task with confidence and skill.

Physicians in a variety of practice settings are tasked with teaching and evaluating students and may be approached to write a letter of recommendation (LOR). Writing an LOR can be a daunting task, especially for those unfamiliar with its expected structure and content. With this article, we provide a framework that any author can use to craft a strong LOR to facilitate a successful application for residency.

LORs are an integral component of residency selection and have been shown to correlate with performance in pediatric internship.[1] They provide an opportunity to highlight applicants' professionalism and adherence to ethical standards, which are qualities important to program directors when selecting applicants to interview.[2] In the next few years, US Medical Licensing Examination Step 1 will transition to a pass-fail test, and residency programs may increasingly rely on other aspects of the application, such as the LOR, to identify candidates that are a good match for their programs.[3]

Despite their importance, concerns have been raised about the lack of standardization of LORs, including variability in their structure, content, and interpretation by faculty.[4,5] One common critique of LORs involves the existence of controversial and unofficial "code words" contained within the letter. For example, "excellent" may be viewed as less favorable than descriptors such as "outstanding" or "one of the best."[6] However, the hierarchy of adjectives is not universal across individuals or institutions. Furthermore, comments intended as positive by letter writers, such as "showed improvement," can be interpreted negatively by letter readers.[7] Therefore, it is important that authors recognize the potential coded language commonly used in LORs to avoid unintentionally harming a student's application with "insufficient" praise.

PREPARE FOR THE LETTER

A conversation with the student provides valuable insight about the student's hopes, goals, and strengths. Asking the student about significant clinical encounters, service activities, or life experiences can help define what they would like to highlight about themselves. Review the student's

[a]Department of Pediatrics, Perelman School of Medicine at the University of Pennsylvania, The Children's Hospital of Philadelphia, Philadelphia, Pennsylvania; [b]Department of Pediatrics, School of Medicine, University of Washington, Seattle, Washington; [c]Department of Pediatrics, School of Medicine, University of South Carolina, Columbia, South Carolina; and [d]Prisma Health Upstate, Greenville, South Carolina

Drs Pete Devon, Burns, and Hartke conceptualized and drafted this article and reviewed and revised the manuscript; and all authors approved the final manuscript as submitted and agree to be accountable for all aspects of the work.

DOI: https://doi.org/10.1542/peds.2020-049615

Accepted for publication Dec 18, 2020

Address correspondence to Erin Pete Devon, MD, The Children's Hospital of Philadelphia, 3401 Civic Center Blvd, Philadelphia, PA 19104. E-mail: petedevone@email.chop.edu

PEDIATRICS (ISSN Numbers: Print, 0031-4005; Online, 1098-4275).

FINANCIAL DISCLOSURE: The authors have indicated they have no financial relationships relevant to this article to disclose.

FUNDING: No external funding.

POTENTIAL CONFLICT OF INTEREST: The authors have indicated they have no potential conflicts of interest to disclose.

To cite: Pete Devon E, Burns R, Hartke A. The LETTER of Recommendation: Showcasing a Student's Strengths. *Pediatrics.* 2021;147(3):e2020049615

curriculum vitae (CV) to learn more about their experiences and accomplishments. The themes and narrative stories that arise from their CV and your conversation will help in writing a compelling LOR.

After meeting with the student, if the author does not think they can write a strong, fair, accurate, or timely letter, this should be disclosed to the student. The student should have the opportunity to seek out another letter writer who can honestly and accurately support their application.

Lastly, as you prepare to write your letter, we encourage new letter writers to contact leaders in the undergraduate or graduate educational program. They may be able to provide examples or guidance on the basis of their experience.

WRITE THE LETTER

To assist letter writers in creating an informative and impactful LOR, we propose the mnemonic "LETTER" as a framework for the important components and their suggested order (see Table 1).

The letter should be concise and ~1 to 2 pages. A particularly short letter may be misconstrued as a bad letter, despite the accolades it highlights. Similarly, a long letter may lose its impact.

Length and Location (Context of Interaction)

Orient the reader to the depth and capacity in which you worked with the student. Briefly describe your role and the rotation or clinical context in which you worked together. This might include the length of the rotation and a brief description of the clinical setting or patient population. If applicable, highlight your experience supervising or teaching medical students, residents, or other medical trainees. These details allow the reader to understand the rigor of the experience and your familiarity with the student's skills, behaviors, and knowledge.

Experience of the Student

Briefly, share the student's role and responsibilities during the rotation. This may include aspects such as patient load, degree of autonomy,

clinical duties, interactions with interprofessional team members, and sensitivity and responsiveness to a diverse patient population.

Traits of the Student

Discuss unique clinical abilities and personal traits of the student that a CV, test scores, and grades do not capture well. Emphasize in what areas a student excels, such as patient care, medical knowledge, communication skills, teamwork, and self-directed learning. Focusing exclusively on nonclinical attributes like punctuality and enthusiasm may lead some readers to believe that other attributes like knowledge, clinical reasoning, or ability to develop rapport with a patient may be lacking, even if that was not your intent. While describing strengths, take care to avoid personal remarks and comments that may reflect bias. For example, avoid commenting on personal appearance or English fluency. Do not use descriptors that may reinforce stereotypes and be mindful of praising effort rather than accomplishment.[8]

TABLE 1 Structuring an LOR

Key Components of an LOR	Helpful Questions to Answer	Example
Length and location	What is the context of your interaction with the student?	I worked with Jenny during the ambulatory portion of her clerkship. In addition to the inpatient responsibilities of that rotation, she worked with me for 3 afternoons each week over the course of 3 weeks in our primary care pediatric practice and assisted in staffing nursery patients after clinic.
Experience of the student	What was the student's experience while working with you?	During the rotation, Jenny functioned in the role of a subintern, independently gathering histories and performing physical examinations under my supervision. Additional responsibilities included providing anticipatory guidance to families.
Traits of the student	What are the student's unique personal and clinical attributes?	Jenny has an outstanding fund of knowledge and can quickly synthesize data to create an accurate assessment and plan.
Tell a story	Share an example to support some of the adjectives you use to describe the student.	I was particularly impressed by her ability to handle a busy room with 2 active toddlers and worried parents with many questions. She was able to distract the toddlers with toys and answer the parents' questions with appropriate confidence.
Educational summary and professional potential	Are there activities or accomplishments from their CV for which you can provide additional context and future application?	Jenny's advocacy experience and community engagement, working to improve access of care to children of recent immigrants demonstrate her dedication to justice. She is poised to have a significant impact on the health and well-being of her patients and community.
Recap	What is your bottom line?	I have supervised medical students and residents for the past 5 years and would rank Jenny among the top X% of all students with whom I have worked. I would be excited to have her remain here for residency.

Tell a Story

Sharing a clinical story that reflects the student's skill sets will captivate a reader's attention more than a laundry list of strengths. A story will paint a broader picture of their clinical and communication skills and professional behaviors.

Educational Summary and Professional Potential

Without repeating the entire CV, describe the student's contributions, and discuss how they reflect the impact the student will have on their patients and their families, the profession, and society in general. Describe how the student will uniquely contribute to their future training program and the education of their peers.

Recap

End the LOR with a summary of highlights of the student and your main message. Summary statements such as "I give my highest recommendation" and "I would recruit this student to stay at our institution/my practice" are statements viewed as most positive by pediatric program directors. Statements including "showed improvement," "performed at expected level," and "solid performance" are viewed as most negative.[9] If possible, summarize a student's attributes compared with the average student with whom you have worked. Truthful phrases such as "in the top 10%" or "one of the best in the past 5 years" help others understand your perspective of their attributes and talents. Remember to be honest. Do not undermine students who are outstanding by giving everyone high remarks.

FINALIZE AND SUBMIT THE LETTER

Once a student submits your name as a letter writer, you will receive an e-mail notification from the Electronic Residency Application Service with instructions. These will include the student's Association of American Medical Colleges identification number, which should be included at the top of the letter. Your final letter should be printed on professional letterhead and include your signature, name and title, and the date. You should include a statement at the bottom of the LOR stating whether the student did or did not waive their right to see the letter. Finally, all letter writers should proofread their letter before submission. Remember, the quality of a letter reflects not only the student but also the writer!

ACKNOWLEDGMENTS

We thank Robert A. Dudas, MD; Michael S. Ryan, MD, MEHP; and Janice L. Hanson, PhD, for their helpful comments and thoughtful reviews of the article.

ABBREVIATIONS

CV: curriculum vitae
LOR: letter of recommendation

REFERENCES

1. Gross C, O'Halloran C, Winn AS, et al. Application factors associated with clinical performance during pediatric internship. *Acad Pediatr.* 2020;20(7): 1007–1012

2. National Resident Matching Program, Data Release and Research Committee. *Results of the 2020 NRMP Program Director Survey.* Washington, DC: National Resident Matching Program; 2020

3. US Medical Licensing Examination. Invitational conference on USLE scoring: change to pass/fail score reporting for Step 1. Available at: https://www.usmle. org/incus/. Accessed December 2, 2020

4. Girzadas DV Jr., Harwood RC, Dearie J, Garrett S. A comparison of standardized and narrative letters of recommendation. *Acad Emerg Med.* 1998;5(11):1101–1104

5. Dirschl DR, Adams GL. Reliability in evaluating letters of recommendation. *Acad Med.* 2000;75(10):1029

6. Morgenstern BZ, Zalneraitis E, Slavin S. Improving the letter of recommendation for pediatric residency applicants: an idea whose time has come? *J Pediatr.* 2003;143(2): 143–144

7. Saudek K, Treat R, Goldblatt M, Saudek D, Toth H, Weisgerber M. Pediatric, surgery, and internal medicine program director interpretations of letters of recommendation. *Acad Med.* 2019;94(11S):S64–S68

8. Turrentine FE, Dreisbach CN, St Ivany AR, Hanks JB, Schroen AT. Influence of gender on surgical residency applicants' recommendation letters. *J Am Coll Surg.* 2019;228(4):356–365.e3

9. Saudek K, Saudek D, Treat R, Bartz P, Weigert R, Weisgerber M. Dear program director: deciphering letters of recommendation. *J Grad Med Educ.* 2018;10(3):261–266

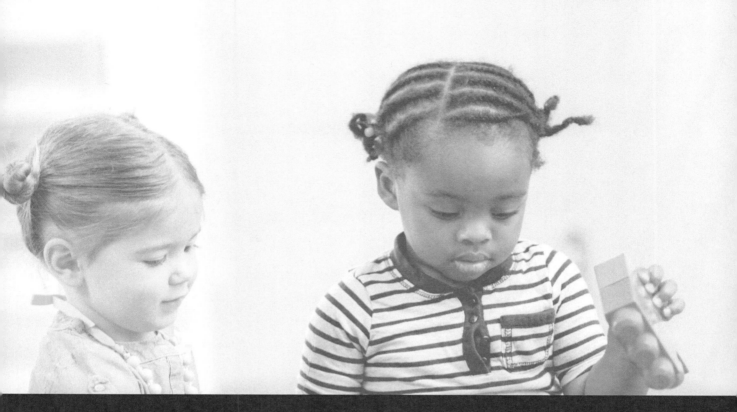

Chapter 5: Clinical Reasoning

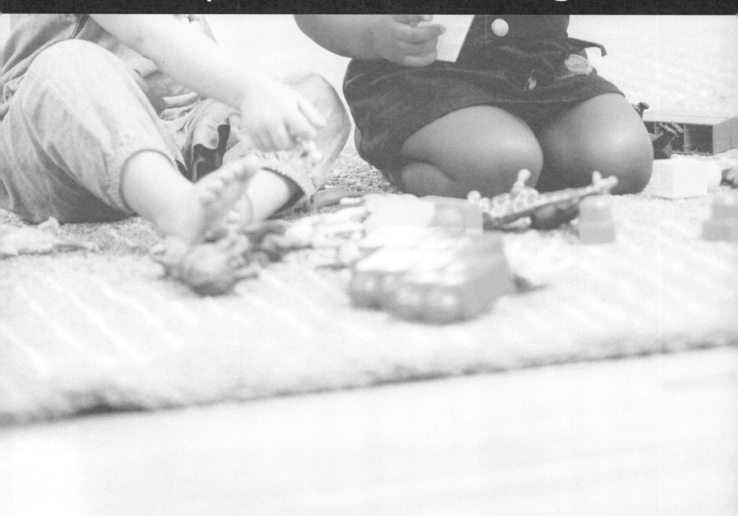

Chapter 5

Promoting Clinical Reasoning and Reflection: The Clinical Teacher as Guide

By Karen L Forbes, MD, MEd, FRCPC
Associate Professor of Pediatrics, Faculty of Medicine & Dentistry, University of Alberta

The breadth of what a student needs to learn in the clinical setting is enormous and often is assumed to occur implicitly. Many cognitively challenging tasks occur during patient interactions including gathering relevant data, synthesizing information, developing an accurate representation of the clinical scenario, and generating and prioritizing an appropriate differential diagnosis, all of which collectively contribute to a clinician's clinical reasoning.[1] Rather than assume that a student tacitly will develop a multitude of skills, this collection of articles suggests concrete strategies to guide students in their learning not only of knowledge, but in developing these skills that are essential in the transition from student to doctor.

A **guide** (n.) is defined as "one who shows the ways to others," and in the active form, **to guide** (v.) is to "direct or have an influence on the course of action of someone or something."[2] Imagine a novice hiker about to embark on an expedition. A guide who has expertise in such experiences may help show "the way" to the hiker by assisting the novice in planning and preparation, directly leading them on their journey, and helping navigate uncertainties, all in an effort to reach the hiker's destination. In clinical educational encounters, the clinician, like the novice hiker's guide, possesses certain expertise and has a role in planning strategies, preparing the learner, and ultimately assisting and showing "the way" to the learner to reach their ultimate goal.

Each of the articles in this chapter highlights a unique opportunity that places the clinical teacher in the role as a student's guide. This expert guidance may be provided at various opportune times, including before the patient encounter, during the student's case presentation, or after the encounter has concluded.

Considering each time point, priming a student before a patient encounter can guide them to obtain relevant data, specific to the clinical context.[3] Following the patient encounter, the student's case presentation provides many opportunities for the clinical teacher to offer guidance. By setting expectations in advance about what is to be included in a case presentation and why,[4] as well as through use of techniques such as the One-Minute Preceptor, SNAPPS,[5] problem representations, and illness scripts among others,[6] the clinical teacher can provide direction on the student's cognitive processes as they learn to think like a doctor. When uncertainties in diagnostic reasoning arise, the clinical teacher can support learners to embrace and address diagnostic challenges.[7] Finally, reflection-in-action and reflection-on-action, the clinical teacher truly can guide the student in their professional identify formation in the domains of doctor as expert, scholar, and person.[8]

Balancing the care of patients with the teaching of learners in a busy clinical setting is one of the most common challenges clinical teachers face. Time constraints abound. The clinical teacher should be reminded that not every technique needs to be implemented for every patient encounter and that a focused approach in guiding the student can be undertaken. Some aspects of guidance, such as laying out expectations for the clinical presentation, may be required only once, whereas others may be used alone or combination with individual clinical encounters. Knowing one's learners and their learning needs may provide the clinical teacher with insight as to what aspects of guidance to focus on.

Considering our novice hiker, the ultimate goal may be reaching the summit of a mountain or arriving at the end of a trail. But the journey does end, and so too may the guide's job. In contrast, our learner's goal may not be singular or as obvious. The journey of the medical student is one of many small hikes in the form of many individual encounters. With each patient encounter, the student constantly is building on previous learning and developing clinical competence. They more efficiently and successfully will do so with the assistance of the clinician teacher, the guide.

References

1. Bowen JL. Educational Strategies to Promote Clinical Diagnostic Reasoning. *NEJM* 2006; 355(21):2217-25.
2. www.dictionary.com accessed 26 June 2020.
3. Stuart E, Hanson JL, Dudas RA. The Right Stuff: Priming Students to Focus on Pertinent Information During Clinical Encounters. *Pediatrics* 2019; 144(1)e20191311.
4. Dell M, Lewin L, Gigante J. What's the Story? Expectations for Oral Case Presentations. *Pediatrics* 2012; 130(1):1-4. DOI:10.1542/peds.2012-1014.
5. Bannister SL, Hanson JL, Maloney, Raszka Jr. WV. Using the Student Case Presentation to
6. Enhance Diagnostic Reasoning. *Pediatrics* 2011; 128(2):211-3. DOI:10.1542/peds.2011-1149.
7. Fleming A Cutrer W, Reimschisel T, Gigante J. You Too Can Teach Clinical Reasoning! *Pediatrics* 2012; 130(5):795-7. DOI:10.1542/peds.2012-2410.
8. Beck JB, Long M, Ryan MS. Into the Unknown: Helping Learners Become More Comfortable with Diagnostic Uncertainty. *Pediatrics* 2020; 146(5)e2020027300. DOI:10.1542/peds.2020-027300.
9. Butani L, Blankenburg R, Long M. Stimulating Reflective Practice Among Your Learners. *Pediatrics* 2013; 131(2): 204-6. DOI:10.1542/peds.2012-3106.

The Right Stuff: Priming Students to Focus on Pertinent Information During Clinical Encounters

Elizabeth Stuart, MD, MSEd,[a] Janice L. Hanson, PhD,[b] Robert Arthur Dudas, MD[c]

Prioritization of relevant information during clinical encounters is a skill that is critical to learn but not easy to teach. In this article, from the Council on Medical Student Education in Pediatrics series on strategies used by great clinical teachers, we offer a framework for coaching students to understand clinical relevance and increase their efficiency in patient care.

THINKING LIKE DOCTORS

Medical students face several challenges when moving from the classroom to the clinical setting. In addition to new roles, responsibilities, and approaches to learning, the transition brings a shift in how students are expected to process and attend to clinical information.[1,2] To work and learn effectively among clinician supervisors, students must move from thinking like students to thinking like doctors.

In particular, students who are new to the clinical setting often notice a change in expectations for history taking, physical examinations, and case presentations. Preclinical training typically encourages a comprehensive, systematic, and formulaic approach to data gathering. As a result, students' early case presentations tend to be highly structured and thorough. Once they enter the time-constrained, practically oriented

clinical setting, students are often asked to streamline, work efficiently, and focus on pertinent details.[3]

A key challenge for clinical teachers is to help students transition their approach. Although the ability to focus on relevant information is one of the most essential elements of medical reasoning and communication, experts have observed that is also one of the most difficult to learn and teach.[2]

LEARNING AND TEACHING WHAT IS PERTINENT

Haber and Lingard[4,5] have looked closely at how students learn to make "relevance decisions" in the context of the development of oral case presentation skills. In observations of inpatient rounds, they noted that supervisors frequently gave students feedback to focus on pertinent or relevant information but rarely defined clinical relevance or provided instruction on how to identify pertinent details. Without explicit guidance, students misinterpreted instructions to streamline their communication, drawing inaccurate conclusions about why specific information was deemed pertinent or not. In the case of a patient with a complicated social history, for example, 1 student interpreted instructions to "Just give me the social context stuff when it's warranted" as an

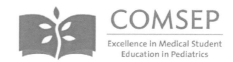

[a]Department of Pediatrics, Stanford School of Medicine, Stanford University, Stanford, California; [b]Office of Education, Washington University School of Medicine in St Louis, St Louis, Missouri; and [c]Department of Pediatrics, Johns Hopkins University School of Medicine, Baltimore, Maryland

Dr Stuart conceptualized and designed this article and drafted, revised, and finalized the manuscript; Drs Hanson and Dudas conceptualized and designed this article, reviewed it critically, and contributed substantially to revisions; and all authors approved the final version to be published and agree to be accountable for all aspects of the work.

DOI: https://doi.org/10.1542/peds.2019-1311

Accepted for publication Apr 24, 2019

Address correspondence to Robert Arthur Dudas, MD, Department of Pediatrics, Johns Hopkins All Children's Hospital, 601 5th St South, Suite 606, St Petersburg, FL 33701. E-mail: rdudas@jhmi.edu

PEDIATRICS (ISSN Numbers: Print, 0031-4005; Online, 1098-4275).

FINANCIAL DISCLOSURE: The authors have indicated they have no financial relationships relevant to this article to disclose.

FUNDING: No external funding.

POTENTIAL CONFLICT OF INTEREST: The authors have indicated they have no potential conflicts of interest to disclose.

To cite: Stuart E, Hanson JL, Dudas RA. The Right Stuff: Priming Students to Focus on Pertinent Information During Clinical Encounters. *Pediatrics.* 2019;144(1):e20191311

TABLE 1 Pre-encounter Priming Examples

Scenarios	Examples of Preceptor Prompts, Coaching	Explanation
• Inexperienced student or student seeing a patient with an unfamiliar problem • Limited time for pre-encounter priming and coaching	• This patient is coming back to clinic for follow-up of ADHD. • Our key goals are to determine if the medication seems to be working as expected and whether there are any side effects. • With those goals in mind, we'll want to review input from the patient, teacher, and parent about attention, behavior, and ability to complete school work. Be sure to ask for the parent and teacher follow-up questionnaires that were given at the last visit. To identify any medication side effects, you'll particularly want to look at growth and ask about changes in appetite or sleep.	Preceptor works through all 3 steps in the framework for the student: • States the key problem • Lists goals for the visit • Explains what key information is needed and how details connect to the broad goals of care.
• More experienced student or student seeing a patient with relatively familiar problem • Time for discussion-based pre-encounter priming and coaching	• This infant is being admitted with a febrile UTI. Tell me what you think should be on his problem list and what our goals should be for managing each problem. • Good. I would add identifying any underlying anatomic predisposition to UTI to our list of goals. • Now, based on your understanding of our goals for this patient, what details do you think are going to be most critical to gather and present?	Preceptor prompts the student to go through all 3 steps in the framework: • Checks the student's understanding of the broad clinical picture (problem list and goals) • Provides feedback on student's ideas for problems and goals. • Coaches student to identify and prioritize pertinent clinical data
• Experienced student, familiar problem, and/or limited time	• When you preround on our patient with bronchiolitis this morning, remember to keep in mind our problem list and the goals for each problem. • Before you see the infant, decide what details are going to be most critical to gather and present on rounds so that we can assess progress and make decisions for each problem and goal.	Preceptor provides a quick reminder or frame. • Articulates steps in the framework • Encourages student to think deliberately about which details are most pertinent to clinical decision-making.

ADHD, attention-deficit/hyperactivity disorder; UTI, urinary tract infection.

idiosyncratic preference of the supervisor ("Some people just don't have an interest in people's social lives…"). The student was later confused when the same supervisor wanted to hear detailed social information as the patient was nearing discharge.[5] When expert clinicians in the study were interviewed, they were unable to articulate a process for determining if a particular detail was relevant. Their understanding of relevance was tacit, intuitive, and therefore difficult to teach. On the basis of these observations, the authors recommended that clinical teachers work deliberately to unpack their tacit understanding, "communicating clearly and repeatedly" to students how the broad context of a medical encounter determines which details are most relevant.[5]

Priming is an educational strategy that offers an opportunity to do just that.

PRIMING STUDENTS TO FOCUS ON PERTINENT INFORMATION: FROM PROBLEMS TO GOALS TO DETAILS

Priming refers to any intervention taken to prepare a learner for an educational experience or task. In the medical education literature, priming typically involves brief coaching just before a patient encounter. It may include telling the student what information to collect, how much time to spend, what the supervisor's role will be, or how information should be presented.[6,7]

Priming can also help students decide what details will be most pertinent to a case. The following problems-goals-details framework for priming is grounded in the idea that relevance is dictated by the goals for the encounter. Of note, although priming can help students judge relevance in the context of diagnostic reasoning, we will focus our attention here on clinical decision-making for patients

with established diagnoses in clinic or on the ward.

The framework emphasizes 3 questions for the student to consider before seeing the patient:

1. What are the patient's problems?

2. What are the goals (established or anticipated) for managing each problem?

3. What details will be most important (pertinent) in assessing progress toward each goal?

For example, in the case of an infant being seen in clinic for suspected viral gastroenteritis, an anticipated problem might be dehydration. A key goal could be articulated as "assess hydration status," and pertinent details would be those that the provider needs to make that assessment (eg, fluid intake and output, change in weight, heart rate, and examination findings reflecting hydration).

Having anticipated which information will be most relevant, on the basis of an understanding of problems and goals, the student reviews the chart and sees the patient, making sure to gather and focus on pertinent details. The case presentation after the encounter emphasizes those same details.

The role of the teacher in priming can be varied according to the student's level of experience, the complexity of the patient, and the amount of time available for coaching. For example, the preceptor can model the process by thinking out loud about problems, goals, and links to pertinent details. Alternatively, the preceptor can question the student about goals and relevant data, or simply provide a reminder to consider context as a guide for how to focus. Table 1 provides examples of these different approaches.

Priming before every clinical encounter is not necessary. Preceptors in the outpatient setting might opt to introduce the problems-goals-details framework at the start of a clinic session and refer back to it when providing feedback during case presentations. Inpatient supervisors might present the framework as a tool for prerounding and planning presentations, either verbally or as a written worksheet that prompts students to articulate problems, goals,

and details. Priming need not occur just before a patient is seen but can involve a brief discussion during downtime to verify students' understanding of their patients' problems, goals, and relevant data.

Regardless of the exact approach taken, students who are primed by using the problems-goals-details framework begin clinical encounters with a mental roadmap that outlines the big picture, with links to relevant data. Priming students in this manner, although it takes a bit of time up front, can increase students' efficiency in seeing patients while helping them build skill in determining clinical relevance.

CONCLUSIONS

Learning to identify and communicate pertinent information is an essential task for clinical learners. Over time, this skill may develop naturally, but it is known to present a challenge. Priming before clinical encounters, with deliberate attention to establishing links between problems, goals, and related details, may enhance learners' gradual progress in making the shift from thinking like a student to thinking like a doctor. Ultimately, empowering students to recognize and focus on pertinent information enables them to align with supervisors' needs, work more

efficiently, and contribute more authentically and meaningfully to patient care.

REFERENCES

1. O'Brien B, Cooke M, Irby DM. Perceptions and attributions of third-year student struggles in clerkships: do students and clerkship directors agree? *Acad Med.* 2007;82(10):970–978

2. Han H, Roberts NK, Korte R. Learning in the real place: medical students' learning and socialization in clerkships at one medical school. *Acad Med.* 2015; 90(2):231–239

3. Dell M, Lewin L, Gigante J. What's the story? Expectations for oral case presentations. *Pediatrics.* 2012;130(1): 1–4

4. Lingard LA, Haber RJ. What do we mean by "relevance"? A clinical and rhetorical definition with implications for teaching and learning the case-presentation format. *Acad Med.* 1999; 74(suppl 10):S124–S127

5. Haber RJ, Lingard LA. Learning oral presentation skills: a rhetorical analysis with pedagogical and professional implications. *J Gen Intern Med.* 2001;16(5):308–314

6. Heidenreich C, Lye P, Simpson D, Lourich M. The search for effective and efficient ambulatory teaching methods through the literature. *Pediatrics.* 2000; 105(1 pt 3):231–237

7. Grover M. Priming students for effective clinical teaching. *Fam Med.* 2002;34(6): 419–420

PEDIATRICS PERSPECTIVES

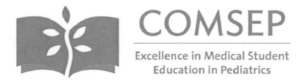

COMSEP

Excellence in Medical Student
Education in Pediatrics

CONTRIBUTORS: Michael Dell, MD,[a] Linda Lewin, MD,[b] and Joseph Gigante, MD[c]

[a]Department of Pediatrics, Case Western Reserve University School of Medicine, Rainbow Babies and Children's Hospital, Cleveland, Ohio; [b]Department of Pediatrics, University of Maryland School of Medicine, Baltimore, Maryland; and [c]Department of Pediatrics, Vanderbilt University School of Medicine, Nashville, Tennessee

Address correspondence to Michael Dell, MD, Department of Pediatrics, Case Western Reserve University School of Medicine, Rainbow Babies and Children's Hospital, 11100 Euclid Ave, Cleveland, OH 44122. E-mail: michael.dell@uhhospitals.org

Accepted for publication Apr 5, 2012

doi:10.1542/peds.2012-1014

What's the Story? Expectations for Oral Case Presentations

This article focuses on teaching and evaluating oral presentation skills as part of the ongoing Council on Medical Student Education in Pediatrics (COMSEP) series on skills and strategies used by superb clinical teachers. While oral presentations by students can be used to enhance diagnostic reasoning,[1] we will focus this article on the characteristics of high-quality oral presentations by medical students, highlight several common pitfalls, and reinforce the connection between effective oral presentations and clinical reasoning. A model for evaluating student clinical performance, the RIME model, will be reviewed.

SETTING EXPECTATIONS

Students often struggle with what is expected of them when asked to give an oral presentation of a patient encounter. Many preceptors have asked a student to present a case, only to be answered with the question, "What would you like to hear?" Students frequently perceive the oral presentation as "a rule-based, data-storage activity governed by order and structure."[2] Clinicians, however, view the oral presentation as a flexible form of communication, with content determined by the clinical context and audience. The first step in bridging this gap is to set explicit expectations. Students should be told early in the clinical experience the commonly accepted and expected style for oral presentations and the rationale for the organization. The ultimate goal of the presentation is to provide the justification for diagnostic and therapeutic decisions. Table 1 summarizes the elements of an effective oral presentation.[3]

ORGANIZATION OF THE EFFECTIVE ORAL PRESENTATION

Chief Complaint: Who Are We Talking About?

Presenting information in an expected order makes it easier for listeners to process information. This begins with the chief complaint. Either a direct quote (eg, "My tummy hurts") or an identifying statement ("A 6-year-old girl with fever and abdominal pain") sets the context for this patient's story from the first line (a different context than that of a 16-year-old girl with abdominal pain!). Most preceptors prefer the latter style, which combines the chief complaint with important demographic and baseline data about the patient.

History of Present Illness: Tell a Good Story

Once the context is set, students should present the history in the order that makes the most sense, bringing in appropriate information from other parts of the history if that information significantly can affect the differential diagnosis. Our thinking about the girl with fever and abdominal pain changes considerably if she had her appendix removed 1 week earlier. However, some students may inappropriately relegate information regarding her surgery to

TABLE 1 Oral Presentation Expectations Checklist[3]

Expectations	Tips for Teaching	Not Done	Needs to Improve	Done Well
Chief complaint	Direct quote from patient or brief identifying statement that includes the patient's age and complaint			
History of present illness	Chronologically organized			
	Tells a clear story			
	Includes pertinent positives and negatives that help distinguish among possible diagnoses			
	Includes elements of past history (such as medications, family history, social history) that specifically contribute to the present illness			
Physical examination	Includes vital signs and general appearance			
	Includes abnormal findings and pertinent elements of physical examination			
Laboratory data	Includes pertinent and/or significant laboratory results/studies			
Summary statement	Synthesizes the critical elements of case into 1 sentence			
	Includes epidemiology (age, gender, ethnicity, race, predisposing conditions)			
	Includes key features (symptoms, physical examination findings, laboratory data)			
	Uses semantic qualifiers			
Assessment	Includes prioritized problem list			
	Includes pertinent differential diagnosis for each problem			
	Identifies most likely diagnosis (and why)			
	Includes less likely diagnoses (and why)			
Plan	Organized by problem list			
	Includes diagnostic plans			
	Includes therapeutic plans			

the past medical history (PMH) because they believe that the "rules" of presentation dictate this. Too often, students abbreviate the history of present illness (HPI) and fail to report the sequence of events, what has made the patient better or worse, the characteristics of the complaint, or associated symptoms.

The Rest of the History

The elements of the PMH, family and social histories, and review of systems that should be included in an oral case presentation depend on the patient's story and the details necessary to help the listener develop a good assessment. This may be difficult for inexperienced students, whose clinical reasoning skills might not yet be sufficiently developed to recognize which details are relevant. A preceptor may ask students to focus on just the "pertinent positives and negatives," yet many students do not understand what this means. Pertinent information helps to answer a question about the patient's illness: What is the diagnosis? How sick is this

patient? Is the patient getting better or worse? For any piece of datum presented, students should be able to explain how that datum contributes to answering a question. A sibling with vomiting and diarrhea is pertinent to our girl with abdominal pain, but less so for another patient with wheezing.

The Physical Examination and Diagnostic Studies

All patient presentations should include the vital signs, the general appearance of the patient, and the key elements of the physical examination. Again, the student should not list all features of the physical examination, only those critical to the diagnosis. In our patient, an expanded report on the abdominal examination and her diffuse abdominal tenderness would be crucial, while a description of normal tympanic membranes should be skipped. A similar rule applies to results of diagnostic studies, which should be reported if relevant to answering 1 of the questions given earlier.

Following the Script

Inexperienced students tend to present information in the order in which it comes to their mind. They may report that "she said that her abdominal pain was severe, but there was no abdominal guarding on my exam," blurring the distinction between history and physical examination findings. Similarly, students may mix objective findings with opinion, such as, "The stool was guaiac negative so bacterial infection seems less likely." Using a written template may help students' organization. From the preceptor's perspective, adherence to the generally accepted organizational structure allows preceptors to more readily identify gaps in data collection.

Summary Statements: The "1-Liner"

Once the history, physical examination, and data are presented, students should summarize the case in 1 or 2 sentences. This summary statement is not a repetition of the identifying statement used at the opening of the presentation.

A good summary statement includes (1) key features, (2) epidemiology, and (3) important qualifying adjectives.

Key features may be symptoms, physical examination findings, or laboratory findings. For our girl with abdominal pain, this would include fever and abdominal pain (identified in the chief complaint), plus any other major symptoms, such as vomiting, diarrhea, and decreased urine output. Key examination findings might include tachycardia, dry mucous membranes, and diffuse abdominal tenderness. Key laboratory data might include a decreased serum bicarbonate level and elevated creatinine level. Key features should be combined into the simplest clinical terms; in this case, oliguria, tachycardia, dry mucous membranes, and elevated creatinine could be synthesized as dehydration.

Epidemiology includes demographics such age (6 years old), gender (girl), and, when pertinent, ethnicity and race. Also included are predisposing conditions (recent appendectomy) and risk factors (sibling with vomiting and diarrhea).

Qualifying adjectives are those that further define key features.[4] These qualifiers serve to identify critical decision points in diagnostic reasoning, such as nonbilious (versus bilious) vomiting, and diffuse (versus localized) abdominal pain. Qualifiers may also describe the progression and severity of illness, such as acute (versus chronic) onset and profuse (versus mild) vomiting.

Pulling it all together, a student who reports that "our patient is a 6-year-old girl status post recent appendectomy, now with acute onset of profuse vomiting and diarrhea associated with diffuse abdominal pain and complicated by severe dehydration" has gone far beyond simply repeating the facts of the preceding presentation and is ready to move on to an assessment.

Assessment: Why Is This Patient Ill?

The assessment should include a rank-ordered discussion of the most likely diagnoses, with arguments in favor of the most likely diagnoses and against less likely possibilities. What is critical is to get students to make a commitment. Novice students tend to offer "laundry lists" of diagnoses in place of a true assessment. Based on the summary statement given earlier, you would expect a student to discuss gastroenteritis and *Clostridium difficile*

infection as possible diagnoses, but a discussion of toxic ingestion or head trauma as causes of vomiting would be unnecessary.

Plan: How Do We Care for This Patient?

Plans should be organized by problem list and subdivided into diagnostic and therapeutic plans. If the cause of our patient's abdominal pain is still in doubt, the plan should propose next steps in evaluation of this problem. For other problems, like our patient's dehydration, the plan will focus on therapeutics.

ASSESSMENT: THE RIME SCHEME

The RIME scheme describes 4 stages of clinical performance: reporter, interpreter, manager and educator.[5] A "reporter" collects data reliably and presents them in an organized fashion. An "interpreter" exhibits clinical reasoning, reporting facts selectively while constructing an argument in the form of an assessment. "Managers" provide diagnostic and therapeutic plans as part of their presentation, while "educators" teach colleagues and patients in a way that uses current experience to enhance future performance and

TABLE 2 RIME Assessment Scheme: Oral Presentations[5]

	Hallmarks of Performance	Barriers to This Level of Achievement
Reporter	Reports reliably	Erroneous details
	Organizes facts	Disorganization
	Collects/reports factual information thoroughly	Missing details
	Answers the "what" questions	
Interpreter	Analyzes data	
	Selectively reports details	Exhaustive report of irrelevant details
	Summarizes case by using descriptive adjectives to describe key features	Case summary only repeats factual details
	Presents a rank-ordered differential diagnoses for this patient	Differential diagnoses presented as nonprioritized list for the chief complaint
	Identifies problem list	No problems identified
	Answers the "why" questions	
Manager/educator	Focuses on decision-making	
	Discusses plans (diagnostic, therapeutic) for each problem	No plan discussed, or plans offered as random "to do" list
	Addresses the issue of "how" to care for patient	
Educator	Educates colleagues through presentations	Cannot explain plan to others
	Discusses patient/family education	Lack of insight/initiation (ie, self-education)
	Identifies topics, resources for self-education	

extrapolates care of the individual patient to broader practice patterns.

The primary goals at the clerkship level are to help students solidify reporting skills and function more consistently at the level of an interpreter. No performance level is beyond the reach of a student, however, and the best students will exhibit manager or educator skills, especially for routine cases. Table 2 summarizes the hallmarks of each level of performance.

CONCLUSIONS

High-quality oral presentations have the potential to promote coordinated patient care, enhance efficiency, and encourage teaching and learning.[6] While the presentation is intended primarily to inform the preceptor about a patient, it also informs the preceptor about the student. High-quality presentations incorporate reliability, organization, clinical reasoning, and decision-making. The RIME scheme provides a useful way to organize observations, which in turn facilitates feedback.

ACKNOWLEDGMENTS

We would like to thank our editors, Susan Bannister, Janice Hanson, and William Raszka, for their helpful comments and thoughtful reviews of the manuscript.

REFERENCES

1. Bannister SL, Hanson JL, Maloney CG, Raszka WV Jr. Using the student case presentation to enhance diagnostic reasoning. *Pediatrics.* 2011;128(2):211–213

2. Haber RJ, Lingard LA. Learning oral presentation skills: a rhetorical analysis with pedagogical and professional implications. *J Gen Intern Med.* 2001;16(5):308–314

3. Lewin LO, Beraho L, Dolan S, Millstein L, Bowman D. Inter-rater reliability of an oral case presentation rating tool in a pediatric clerkship. *Teach Learn Med.* 2012, In press

4. Chang RW, Bordage G, Connell KJ. The importance of early problem representation during case presentations. *Acad Med.* 1998; 73(suppl 10):S109–S111

5. Pangaro L. A new vocabulary and other innovations for improving descriptive in-training evaluations. *Acad Med.* 1999;74(11): 1203–1207

6. Green EH, Hershman W, DeCherrie L, Greenwald J, Torres-Finnerty N, Wahi-Gururaj S. Developing and implementing universal guidelines for oral patient presentation skills. *Teach Learn Med.* 2005;17(3):263–267

FINANCIAL DISCLOSURE: *The authors have indicated they have no financial relationships relevant to this article to disclose.*
FUNDING: No external funding.

PEDIATRICS PERSPECTIVES

CONTRIBUTORS: Susan L. Bannister, MD,[a] Janice L. Hanson, PhD, EdS,[b] Christopher G. Maloney, MD, PhD,[c] and William V. Raszka Jr, MD[d]

[a]Department of Pediatrics, Faculty of Medicine, University of Calgary, Calgary, Alberta, Canada; Departments of [b]Medicine and Pediatrics, Uniformed Services University of the Health Sciences, Bethesda, Maryland; [c]Department of Pediatrics, University of Utah, Salt Lake City, Utah; and [d]Department of Pediatrics, University of Vermont College of Medicine, Burlington, Vermont

Address correspondence to Susan L. Bannister, MD, Department of Pediatrics, Faculty of Medicine, University of Calgary, 2888 Shaganappi Trail NW, Calgary, Alberta, Canada T3B 6A8. E-mail: susan.bannister@albertahealthservices.ca

Accepted for publication May 19, 2011

The views expressed in this article are those of the authors and not necessarily those of the Uniformed Services University of the Health Sciences or the US Department of Defense.

ABBREVIATION
OMP—One-Minute Preceptor

doi:10.1542/peds.2011-1469

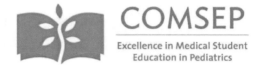

COMSEP
Excellence in Medical Student
Education in Pediatrics

Using the Student Case Presentation to Enhance Diagnostic Reasoning

This article resumes the series by the Council on Medical Student Education in Pediatrics (COMSEP) examining the skills and strategies of great clinical teachers.

So far we have reviewed what makes a clinical teacher great[1] and the importance of orientation,[2] observation,[3] and feedback.[4] In this article we discuss how best to use the time during or after a student case presentation to assess and strengthen student diagnostic reasoning skills. The development of good clinical reasoning skills is an essential component of medical school training and remains critical to clinical practice.

Each of us has heard lengthy presentations from medical students on patients they have seen. The presentations tend to emphasize the facts of the case (the history and what others have done) but often do not include an assessment or any explanation of why the student has come to a particular

conclusion. Using case presentations as a platform, we present 2 models for assessing diagnostic reasoning skills: one in which the student presents the case and drives the learning (SNAPPS)[5] and one in which the preceptor directs the learning by asking 5 types of questions after listening to the case presentation (One-Minute Preceptor [OMP]).[6] Both models are designed for use in a busy office setting with minimal time commitment by the preceptor.

THE SNAPPS MODEL

SNAPPS is a learner-driven model in which the student articulates both his or her diagnostic reasoning processes and uncertainties about the clinical case.[7] SNAPPS stands for "summarize the history and physical findings," "narrow down the differential diagnosis," "analyze the differential," "probe the preceptor about uncertainties," "plan management for the patient," and "select case-related issues for self-study"[5] (see Table 1).

In the SNAPPS model, the student first summarizes the salient features of the case. The summary should be short and directed and should not exceed 50% of the time allotted to the total presentation. The next step for the student is to narrow the differential diagnosis to the 2 or 3 most likely possibilities. This is not an exercise to generate an exhaustive differential, most of which is unlikely. For example, for an 8-year-old with a remote history of asthma and a cough for 1 week, the differential could include asthma exacerbation, viral lower respiratory tract illness, and bacterial pneumonia. The student next analyzes his or her own differential by comparing and contrasting the possibilities or justifying selection of the most likely possibility. In this case, viral illness may be likely, because the student heard no wheezing and there was no environmental trigger. The student next asks the pre-

TABLE 1 Comparison of SNAPPS and the OMP

	SNAPPS	OMP
Driven by	Student	Preceptor
Relation to case presentation	This is the case presentation	Follows the case presentation
No. of steps	6	5
Steps	1. Summarize the case	1. Get a commitment: "What do
	2. Narrow the differential diagnosis	you think is going on with
	3. Analyze the differential	this patient?"
	4. Probe the preceptor about	2. Probe for evidence: "How did
	uncertainties	you reach that conclusion?"
	5. Plan management for the patient	3. Teach 1 to 2 general rules
	6. Select case-related issues for	that will apply to other
	self-study	situations
		4. Reinforce what was done well
		5. Correct mistakes
Ways to make it work	Orient everyone	Orient everyone
	Cards	Cards
	Posters	Posters
	Keep track of learning topics	Keep track of learning topics

ceptor questions about any uncertainties or difficulties he or she may have experienced. Going back to our example, the student might ask the preceptor whether children with asthma exacerbations always present with wheezing. The SNAPPS model differs from most other models used in medical student education, because it specifically supports students in their expression of uncertainty or diagnostic confusion.

Once the student has identified areas of uncertainty, he or she begins a discussion about how to manage the patient. Because this is in the context of direct patient care, the student cannot waffle using words such as "might" and "could." Finally, the student identifies, with the help of the preceptor, case-related topics for further study. Importantly, the student commits to a plan to remediate gaps in knowledge or reasoning skills identified during the patient encounter.[7] Because this process is student-directed and built on self-reflection, it is likely to be more powerful than teacher-directed reading.[8]

The SNAPPS model assumes that the primary role of the preceptor is that of

coach or facilitator. The preceptor may teach the model on the first day but thereafter listens to the case presentation, encourages students to complete all components of the process, answers questions, assists in selecting areas for further development, and provides feedback. Videos at www. practicalprof.ab.ca ("teaching nuts and bolts") demonstrate how to use SNAPPS in the office setting.[9]

Although quite different from traditional presentation models, faculty preceptors have required little training in the use of SNAPPS. In a pilot study, the preceptors were merely reminded by telephone that the students would be using the SNAPPS methodology and to encourage its continued use.[5] In another study the preceptors were given a 20-minute orientation on SNAPPS.[7] SNAPPS remains an efficient way to learn about both the patient and the student. The length of the student presentations using SNAPPS, approximately 5 minutes, did not differ significantly from the length of traditional presentations.[7]

Compared with students using a traditional presentation model, students using SNAPPS were more likely to include a differential diagnosis, compare and con-

trast diagnoses, formulate a management plan, and identify topics for further discussion.[7] Also, students enjoy the active learning inherent in the SNAPPS model.[7] SNAPPS allows students to move beyond simple reporting to actively managing patients.

THE OMP MODEL

Similar to the SNAPPS model, the OMP uses the student case presentation as a springboard for assessing and remediating student diagnostic reasoning. However, in contrast to SNAPPS, the OMP model is a 5-step preceptor-driven model[6] (Table 1).

The student begins by presenting the salient features of the case. Once the student has finished the presentation, the first task of the preceptor is to ask the student to commit to a diagnosis or management plan. Once the student has committed, the preceptor probes the student for the supporting evidence used to make the diagnosis or management plan. These 2 steps are key to evaluating student knowledge and reasoning. A practical way to remember the first 2 steps is to ask students "what" is going on and "why." Using our example, the student may state that he or she thinks the patient has a bacterial rather than a viral lung infection because the patient has a fever. Armed with information about both the patient and the student, the preceptor can then teach to general points that can be used in future patient encounters. In this example, the preceptor could briefly state that both viral and bacterial lung infections can lead to fever and that a better finding suggesting a bacterial infection would be the presence of localized crackles. The final steps in the OMP model involve reinforcing what the student has done well, correcting errors, and making recommendations for improvement. Videos that demonstrate effective questions and the OMP model can be viewed at www.practicalprof.ab.ca ("teaching nuts and bolts").[9]

The OMP model has been incorporated successfully into a variety of clinical venues[10,11] and has been shown to improve key teaching behaviors.[10,12,13] The model is not intended to be prescriptive but, rather, a set of guidelines that can be altered to fit the clinical and teaching situation.[14]

CONCLUSIONS

Both SNAPPS and the OMP allow preceptors to assess the diagnostic reasoning skills of learners. Their use can be facilitated by orientation of the student, use of laminated pocket cards to help remember the steps, posters on the wall, and both students and preceptors keeping track of student self-study topics.[15] Using these models allows preceptors to diagnose 2 things: the patient's problem and the student's understanding of the patient's problem. Understanding both of these things is crucial for effective patient care and great clinical teaching.

REFERENCES

1. Bannister SL, Raszka WV Jr, Maloney CG. What makes a great clinical teacher in pediatrics? Lessons learned from the literature. *Pediatrics*. 2010;125(5):863–865

2. Raszka WV Jr, Maloney CG, Hanson JL. Getting off to a good start: discussing goals and expectations with medical students. *Pediatrics*. 2010;126(2):193–195

3. Hanson JL, Bannister SL, Clark A, Raszka WV Jr. Oh, what you can see: the role of observation in medical student education. *Pediatrics*. 2010;126(5):843–845

4. Gigante J, Dell M, Sharkey A. Getting beyond "good job": how to give effective feedback. *Pediatrics*. 2011;127(2):205–207

5. Wolpaw TM, Wolpaw DR, Papp KK. SNAPPS: a learner-centered model for outpatient education. *Acad Med*. 2003;78(9):893–898

6. Neher JO, Gordon KC, Meyer B, Stevens N. A five-step "microskills" model of clinical teaching. *J Am Board Fam Pract*. 1992;5(4):419–424

7. Wolpaw T, Papp KK, Bordage G. Using SNAPPS to facilitate the expression of clinical reasoning and uncertainties: a randomized clinical trial. *Acad Med*. 2009;84(4):517–524

8. Pangaro L. A new vocabulary and other innovations for improving descriptive in-training evaluations. *Acad Med*. 1999;74(11):1203–1207

9. Alberta Rural Physician Action Plan. Key features of great clinical teachers. Available at: www.practicalprof.ab.ca/teaching_nuts_bolts/key_features.html. Accessed May 16, 2011

10. Furney SL, Orsini AN, Orsetti KE, Stern DT, Gruppen GP, Irby DM. Teaching the One-Minute Preceptor: a randomized controlled trial. *J Gen Intern Med*. 2001;16(9):620–624

11. Ferenchick G, Simpson D, Blackman J, DaRosa D, Dunnington G. Strategies for efficient and effective teaching in the ambulatory care setting. *Acad Med*. 1997;72(4):277–280

12. Salerno SM, O'Malley PG, Pangaro LN, Wheeler GA, Moores LK, Jackson JL. Faculty development seminars based on the One-Minute Preceptor improve feedback in the ambulatory setting. *J Gen Intern Med*. 2002;17(10):779–787

13. Aagaard E, Teherani A, Irby DM. Effectiveness of the One-Minute Preceptor model for diagnosing the patient and the learner: proof of concept. *Acad Med*. 2004;79(1):42–49

14. Neher JO, Stevens NG. The One-Minute Preceptor: shaping the teaching conversation. *Fam Med*. 2003;35(6):391–393

15. Centre for Evidence-Based Medicine Toronto. Educational prescriptions. Available at: www.cebm.utoronto.ca/practise/formulate/eduprescript.htm. Accessed May 16, 2011

FINANCIAL DISCLOSURE: *The authors have indicated they have no financial relationships relevant to this article to disclose.*

PEDIATRICS PERSPECTIVES

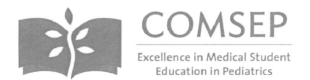

COMSEP
Excellence in Medical Student
Education in Pediatrics

CONTRIBUTORS: Amy Fleming, MD, William Cutrer, MD, MEd, Tyler Reimschisel, MD, and Joseph Gigante, MD
Department of Pediatrics, Vanderbilt University School of Medicine, Nashville, Tennessee

Address correspondence to Joseph Gigante, MD, Department of Pediatrics, Vanderbilt University School of Medicine, 8232 Doctor's Office Tower, Nashville, TN 37232-9225. E-mail: joseph.gigante@vanderbilt.edu

Accepted for publication Aug 20, 2012

ABBREVIATIONS
HSP—Henoch-Schonlein Purpura
RLQ—right lower quadrant

doi:10.1542/peds.2012-2410

You Too Can Teach Clinical Reasoning!

As part of the ongoing Council on Medical Student Education in Pediatrics series on skills and strategies used by great clinical teachers,[1–6] this article focuses on practical knowledge and skills for teaching clinical reasoning. Building on SNAPPS and One Minute Preceptor models,[6] we will address the clinical assessment portion of oral and written presentations that represents the culmination of the clinical reasoning process. Using the concepts of problem representation,[7] semantic qualifiers,[8] and illness scripts[7,9,10] defined below, we will outline how you can guide your students' clinical reasoning development.

PROBLEM REPRESENTATION AND SEMANTIC QUALIFIERS

A problem representation is "the one-liner" at the end of a presentation that synthesizes the entire patient story (history details, physical findings, and investigations) into 1 "big picture" statement.[7] To create a problem representation, physicians restructure pertinent patient details into abstract terms called semantic qualifiers. Semantic qualifiers are abstractions in medical rather than lay terminology and generally exist in divergent pairs, such as acute versus chronic and severe versus mild (Table 1, step 2).[8] Here is an example of a problem representation, with the semantic qualifiers in italics: *A previously well, 2-year-old unimmunized girl presents with an acute history of respiratory distress. She is febrile, looks unwell, and is drooling.*

TEACHING HOW TO ARTICULATE PROBLEM REPRESENTATIONS BY USING SEMANTIC QUALIFIERS

Novice clinicians can be taught to generate problem representations by using semantic qualifiers. First, have your students write out a 1- to 2-sentence problem representation (summary of patient information) based on either a written case or a real patient they have seen. Second, ask them to replace as many details as possible by using semantic qualifiers (Table 1, steps 1–3). Remind them that semantic qualifiers usually come in opposing pairs. For example:

First Draft of a Problem Representation:

The patient is a 16-year-old boy with a history of 2 ear infections who presents with 3 days of fever and abdominal pain that started with dull pain in the periumbilical region and moved to the right lower quadrant (RLQ) with 10/10 pain on the day of admission, 2 days of decreased food intake, and 1 day of vomiting. The physical examination revealed abdominal tenderness, rebound tenderness, and guarding, and the white blood cell count was 20 000.

Rather than making an assessment, the details of the case in this example are merely restated. When semantic qualifiers are used, 2 ear infections becomes "otherwise well," 3 days becomes "acute," and decreased food intake becomes "anorexia," and the key findings of history, physical examination, and laboratories are synthesized to offer the most plausible diagnosis.

TABLE 1 Teaching Steps for Clinical Reasoning

Step 1: Student Presents the Data About a Patient.

Example: The patient is a 16-y-old boy with a history of 2 ear infections who presents with 3 d of fever and abdominal pain. The pain was initially dull and in the peri-umbilical region but is now right sided and 10/10 pain. He has vomited twice and has not eaten anything for 2 d.

Step 2: Discuss Relevant Semantic Qualifiers.

Teaching Questions	Examples of Semantic Qualifiers	
Which medical descriptors apply to this patient?	Acute	Chronic
	Severe	Mild
	Localized	Diffuse
	Previously healthy	Significant past medical history
	Right sided	Left sided

Step 3: Construct a Problem Representation That Incorporates Semantic Qualifiers.

Example: The patient is an *otherwise well* 16-y-old *boy* who presents with *acute* onset of fever, *severe*, *localized*, abdominal pain, vomiting, and anorexia.

Step 4: Compare Illness Scripts for the Most Likely Diagnoses (eg, appendicitis and gastroenteritis).

Teaching Questions	Appendicitis	Acute Gastroenteritis
Predisposing Condition:	Predisposing Condition:	Predisposing Condition:
What epidemiologic factors influence the probability that a patient is at risk for disease (eg, age, gender, past medical history, and environmental influences)?	• no clear predisposing factors	• sick contacts • overseas travel
Pathophysiologic Insult:	Pathophysiologic Insult:	Pathophysiologic Insult:
What are the major pathophysiologic insults that contribute to the disease state?	• fecalith • ischemia of bowel wall • local inflammation • perforation	• effacement of villi • Viral or bacterial invasion • local inflammation
Clinical Consequences:	Clinical Consequences:	Clinical Consequences:
What are the symptoms and signs that may result from the predisposing condition or pathophysiologic insult?	• severe, localized pain • nausea, vomiting, anorexia, diarrhea • fever	• mild, diffuse pain • nausea, vomiting, anorexia, diarrhea • fever +/−

Step 5: Select the Illness Script That Best Matches the Patient's Presentation.

This patient's presentation is most consistent with acute appendicitis.

Revised Draft of Problem Representation:

The patient is an *otherwise well* 16-year-old *boy* who presents with *acute* onset of *fever, severe, localized* abdominal pain, *vomiting*, and *anorexia*. The physical examination and laboratories were significant for *right lower* quadrant pain, *guarding, rebound tenderness*, and an *elevated* white blood cell count. This patient's presentation is most consistent with acute appendicitis.

ILLNESS SCRIPTS

Unlike problem representations and semantic qualifiers that are concrete, the concept of illness scripts is abstract. Illness scripts are what experienced physicians unconsciously use when they assess and diagnose a patient; they are based on real patient experiences, and contain extensive clinically relevant information about how diseases present but few pathophysiological data.[7,9,10] They are structured in our brains,

whether we know it or not, as predisposing condition, pathophysiologic insult, and clinical consequences.[7,9,10]

After hearing a chief complaint, expert clinicians engage in a process of script search, script selection, and script verification.[10] They begin by creating a working differential diagnosis and accessing multiple illness scripts from past clinical experience. Then, they gather further data and explore discriminating features between illness scripts comparing and contrasting their patient with numerous other patients they have seen in the past. Finally, they select the most appropriate illness script and create a working diagnosis. All of this often happens in seconds or minutes and occurs without the physician's conscious thought so that when the student asks "How did you know that so fast?", he or she may be unable to answer.

Here is an example of accessing an illness script. Read each line below to determine when you are fairly confident you know the diagnosis.

1. 16-year-old boy.
2. Admitted for acute abdominal pain.
3. Has poor PO intake.
4. Pain started around his umbilicus but has moved to the RLQ.
5. Febrile to 39.4°C.
6. Has associated nausea, vomiting, and anorexia.

We imagine that many of you reached number 4 and felt confident the diagnosis is appendicitis. Why? Because you accessed the illness script for appendicitis, and you started with 2 or 3 illness scripts after reading the first 3 statements (perhaps acute gastroenteritis, appendicitis, or inflammatory bowel disease). The movement of pain from peri-umbilical to RLQ helped you choose the appendicitis illness script, and further information about fever, anorexia, and nausea reinforced your choice. If we had given you a 16-year-old girl, you would still be comparing the illness scripts for pelvic inflammatory disease or ectopic pregnancy and would need further information to narrow down the appropriate illness script.

Let's repeat this process with a more pediatric-specific diagnosis:

1. 8-year-old boy
2. Admitted for acute abdominal pain
3. Has poor PO intake for the past day
4. Has a purpuric rash in a waist-down distribution
5. Presents with large joint pain
6. Has proteinuria on urinalysis

Note both cases start in similar ways suggesting similar illness scripts (appendicitis, gastroenteritis), yet when pediatricians reach number 4, they change to the illness script of Henoch-Schonlein Purpura (HSP). The purpuric rash described does not match the initial 2 illness scripts and instead correlates with HSP. Joint pain and proteinuria reinforce the HSP illness script. Try this with your nonpediatric colleagues and the second case will be a challenge (they understandably do not recall the illness script for HSP). If you possess the appropriate illness scripts, the process is quick and typically accurate. Trainees, in contrast, have only a few illness scripts, and therefore usually rely on deliberately analyzing case details to determine the diagnosis.

TEACHING HOW TO COMPARE AND CONTRAST ILLNESS SCRIPTS

Although the concept of illness scripts can and should be explained to students, we cannot build their illness scripts for them (they must be constructed by each learner based on the patients they have seen).[9] What we can do is maximize clinical experiences, suggest students read approximately 2 diagnoses at the same time and compare and contrast their similar and discriminating features,[7] and encourage them to articulate the 3 components of an illness script: predisposing conditions, pathophysiolgic insults, and clinical consequences. Table 1, step 4, outlines a process for teaching by using illness scripts.

POTENTIAL PITFALLS OF ILLNESS SCRIPTS

Although illness scripts usually point an experienced clinician to the correct diagnoses, errors do occur. Discussing the types of errors that happen enhances the process of student clinical reasoning development. Errors include fixating on a specific clinical feature too soon in the clinical encounter (anchoring bias), settling on a given diagnosis before fully examining other options (premature closure), and interpreting information so that it supports a previous conclusion (confirmation bias).[11]

CONCLUSIONS

Great clinical teachers recognize the challenge that students face in synthesizing the details of patient information into concise, accurate clinical assessments. We can help by teaching students to articulate clear problem representations by using semantic qualifiers and to compare and contrast their patients with similar cases to develop accurate illness scripts.

ACKNOWLEDGMENTS

We greatly appreciate the thoughtful input and editing from Janice Hanson, Chris Maloney, Susan Bannister, and Bill Raszka.

REFERENCES

1. Raszka WV Jr, Maloney CG, Hanson JL. Getting off to a good start: discussing goals and expectations with medical students. *Pediatrics*. 2010;126(2):193–195

2. Hanson JL, Bannister SL, Clark A, Raszka WV Jr. Oh, what you can see: the role of observation in medical student education. *Pediatrics*. 2010;126(5):843–845

3. Gigante J, Dell M, Sharkey A. Getting beyond "Good job": how to give effective feedback. *Pediatrics*. 2011;127(2):205–207

4. Dell M, Lewin L, Gigante J. What's the story? Expectations for oral case presentations. *Pediatrics*. 2012;130(1):1–4

5. Bannister SL, Raszka WV Jr, Maloney CG. What makes a great clinical teacher in pediatrics? Lessons learned from the literature. *Pediatrics*. 2010;125(5):863–865

6. Bannister SL, Hanson JL, Maloney CG, Raszka WV Jr. Using the student case presentation to enhance diagnostic reasoning. *Pediatrics*. 2011;128(2):211–213

7. Bowen JL. Educational strategies to promote clinical diagnostic reasoning. *N Engl J Med*. 2006;355(21):2217–2225

8. Bordage G. Why did I miss the diagnosis? Some cognitive explanations and educational implications. *Acad Med*. 1999;74 (suppl 10):S138–S143

9. Charlin B, Tardif J, Boshuizen HPA. Scripts and medical diagnostic knowledge: theory and applications for clinical reasoning instruction and research. *Acad Med*. 2000;75 (2):182–190

10. Schmidt HG, Norman GR, Boshuizen HP. A cognitive perspective on medical expertise: theory and implication. [published erratum appears in Acad Med 1992 Apr;67(4):287] *Acad Med*. 1990;65(10):611–621

11. Croskerry P. Achieving quality in clinical decision making: cognitive strategies and detection of bias. *Acad Emerg Med*. 2002;9 (11):1184–1204

FINANCIAL DISCLOSURE: *The authors have indicated they have no financial relationships relevant to this article to disclose.*
FUNDING: No external funding.

Into the Unknown: Helping Learners Become More Comfortable With Diagnostic Uncertainty

Jimmy B. Beck, MD, MEd,[a,b] Michele Long, MD,[c,d] Michael S. Ryan, MD, MEHP[e,f]

A diagnosis is a judgement characterized by uncertainty and probabilistic reasoning: it is seldom definitive at the initial point of care.

Gurpreet Dhaliwal, MD

CLINICAL UNCERTAINTY AND THE IMPACT ON LEARNERS

Great clinical teachers recognize that uncertainty is an inherent aspect of making a clinical diagnosis, particularly when symptoms are nonspecific or change over time. In a recent review, diagnostic uncertainty was defined as a "subjective perception of an inability to provide an accurate explanation of the patient's health problem."[1] Physician discomfort with uncertainty has been associated with burnout, over-testing, increased health care expenditures, and diagnostic errors.[2,3] Over time, skilled clinicians become increasingly comfortable with accepting and navigating uncertainty, in part because they treat diagnoses as provisional hypotheses or "working diagnoses" instead of definitive diagnoses.[4,5] They recognize that clinical reasoning in the face of uncertainty requires a thought process in which several potential diagnoses are weighed as new information is considered, evaluated, and contextualized.[6]

Learners commonly struggle when they encounter uncertainty.[7]

Several reasons may contribute to the difficulty experienced by learners, including limited situation-specific knowledge, fewer relevant previous clinical experiences, lack of formal curricula to address uncertainty, testing strategies that highlight only a single best answer, discomfort sharing uncertainty for fear it will be perceived as weakness or will influence their evaluations,[8] and lack of role models who exemplify approaches for addressing uncertainty.[3]

The ability to accept uncertainty is recognized as a skill that all pediatric residents must demonstrate during their training,[9] yet there are few interventions to prepare medical students and residents to deal with uncertainty.[8,10] Given the harms of discomfort with uncertainty (eg, burnout and over-testing), learning to recognize and process uncertainty is crucial not only for students' own growth but also for the health of their future patients.

GUIDING STUDENTS INTO THE UNKNOWN: SET THE STAGE FOR THE LEARNER AND THE EDUCATOR

Learners may enter clerkships with a notion that diagnoses are always clear, and many believe that when a certain degree of clinical competence has been obtained (such as completing residency), uncertainty will go away. It is

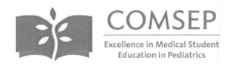

[a]*Department of Pediatrics, University of Washington, Seattle, Washington;* [b]*Seattle Children's Hospital, Seattle, Washington;* [c]*Department of Pediatrics, School of Medicine, University of California, San Francisco, San Francisco, California;* [d]*University of California, San Francisco Benioff Children's Hospital, San Francisco, California;* [e]*Department of Pediatrics, School of Medicine, Virginia Commonwealth University, Richmond, Virginia; and* [f]*Children's Hospital of Richmond at Virginia Commonwealth University, Richmond, Virginia*

Dr Beck conceptualized and designed the manuscript, wrote the initial version, and reviewed and revised the manuscript; Dr Long helped with the conceptualization and design of the manuscript and reviewed and revised the manuscript; Dr Ryan helped with the conceptualization and design of the manuscript, was the primary author of the table, and reviewed and revised the manuscript; and all authors approved the final manuscript as submitted and agree to be accountable for all aspects of the work.

DOI: https://doi.org/10.1542/peds.2020-027300

Accepted for publication Aug 20, 2020

Address correspondence to Jimmy B. Beck, MD, MEd, Seattle Children's Hospital, 4800 Sandpoint Way NE, Mailstop FA.2.115, PO Box 5371, Seattle, WA 98105. E-mail: jimmy.beck@seattlechildrens.org

PEDIATRICS (ISSN Numbers: Print, 0031-4005; Online, 1098-4275).

FINANCIAL DISCLOSURE: The authors have indicated they have no financial relationships relevant to this article to disclose.

FUNDING: No external funding.

POTENTIAL CONFLICT OF INTEREST: The authors have indicated they have no potential conflicts of interest to disclose.

To cite: Beck JB, Long M, Ryan MS. Into the Unknown: Helping Learners Become More Comfortable With Diagnostic Uncertainty. *Pediatrics.* 2020;146(5):e2020027300

therefore crucial that educators normalize uncertainty, when appropriate, in the same way they need to normalize making mistakes.[11] As new pieces of history, examination findings, or diagnostic results emerge, new uncertainties will also emerge. Expert clinical teachers can encourage a growth mindset[12] and can role model habits of lifelong learning because even seasoned clinicians are aware that years of clinical experience still does not "protect against the challenges of uncertainty."[13] As part of orientation, great clinical teachers can talk to learners about the ubiquity of uncertainty in medicine. Using scripts (such as, "Making a diagnosis is sometimes challenging, and often times there are several possibilities that we may need to consider") can help open a dialogue about uncertainty with learners up front.

GUIDING LEARNERS TO ADDRESS UNCERTAINTY WITH THE 1-MINUTE UNCERTAINTY PRECEPTOR

Once the stage is set that discussing uncertainty is not only acceptable but encouraged, the learner now can be taught how to recognize and respond appropriately to this uncertainty. We have adapted a previously described teaching model, the one-minute preceptor, which can serve as a framework for clinical teachers to help learners recognize and respond to uncertainty. The one-minute uncertainty preceptor is outlined in the following section.

First described by Neher et al,[14] the one-minute preceptor is a well-established strategy for clinical teaching that has been shown to improve skills in the domains of medical knowledge and clinical reasoning. The model includes 5 steps: (1) get a commitment, (2) probe for supporting evidence, (3) teach general rules, (4) reinforce what was done well, and (5) correct mistakes. With a few simple modifications to steps 1, 2, and 3, the one-minute preceptor can be adapted to the one-minute uncertainty preceptor to help facilitate targeted conversations regarding uncertainty (Table 1).

Step 1: Commitment and Certainty

This first step allows the educator to identify potential uncertainty in the learner. The traditional one-minute preceptor model requires the learner to commit to a diagnosis or management option. The one-minute uncertainty preceptor incorporates this approach with an additional follow-up question: "How certain are you?" This simple question may help to initiate the conversation between the learner and the educator regarding the relative certainty surrounding a case. Although not all learners will realize they are uncertain or be willing to admit they are uncertain, this opening question can provide an invitation to begin this discussion.

Step 2: Probe for Evidence

This step promotes self-reflection and remains similar to the traditional model but with a specific focus on reasons for the learner's uncertainty. Uncertainty provides an excellent opportunity for reflection. Studies suggest that clinicians who engage in self-reflection can reduce the negative impacts of uncertainty on patient care.[15] In this step, the educator asks the learner to explain the aspects of the case that make them more or less certain so that the educator can facilitate learning focused on uncertainty.

To do this, educators can have learners identify the most disconcerting or the key area(s) that are contributing to their uncertainty. The educator may also ask the learners to discuss other potential diagnoses, how they can mitigate some of the uncertainty, and how they may know if they made the right decision as time passes.

Step 3: Teaching Points and Role Modeling

Finally, the educator can role model an approach to handling uncertainty. In the traditional model, this step

TABLE 1 The One-Minute Uncertainty Preceptor

Step	Description	Example Scripts
1	Commitment and certainty	"What do you think is going on?" "How certain are you?"
2	Probe	"What are the aspects of the case that make you feel more or less certain?" "What else could it be?" "How are you feeling about this case right now?" "What other pieces of information would you want to gather?" "How are you going to monitor whether you made the right decision?" "How are you going to monitor this problem as it progresses?" "What cues might signal that you are veering into dangerous territory when you need help?" "Whom could you call for help?"
3	Teach and role model	"This is how I'm feeling about the case right now." "This is how I weigh the pros and cons in a situation like this." "One way we can tell if we made the right decision is ____." "I'm feeling a little uneasy right now because____." "I'm feeling uncertain of what to do for this patient." "I can't explain why this patient is having bloody stools, but my working hypothesis is____." "You know what my 'unknowns' are for this case…? Given that, here is my action plan."
4	Reinforce what was done well	What the learner did well
5	Correct mistakes	What the learner can do better

allows the educator to highlight 2 to 3 key teaching points based on the case. To modify this step for uncertainty, rather than teach knowledge-based concepts, the educator can address specific aspects of the case that are leading to uncertainty. For example, the educator can call out reasons why one may be uncertain in a situation such as the current case, ways in which one may mitigate that uncertainty, and ways in which one would know if the decision made for a patient was the most appropriate. This step provides an opportunity for the educator to share how he or she leverages discomfort to inform clinical reasoning around an ill-defined problem.

Steps 4 and 5

These steps (reinforce what was done well and correct mistakes) remain unchanged in the one-minute uncertainty preceptor model.

CULTIVATING A LEARNING ENVIRONMENT THAT ACKNOWLEDGES AND EMBRACES UNCERTAINTY

Great clinical teachers can use the one-minute uncertainty preceptor to guide their one-on-one interactions with learners. Equally important, however, is having the educator facilitate an environment that accepts and even embraces diagnostic uncertainty. In this way, the presence of uncertainty is not a reflection of a learner's failure or a demonstration of weakness but rather a welcomed part of clinical reasoning that spurs curiosity, learning, and growth.

REFERENCES

1. Bhise V, Rajan SS, Sittig DF, Morgan RO, Chaudhary P, Singh H. Defining and measuring diagnostic uncertainty in medicine: a systematic review. *J Gen Intern Med*. 2018;33(1):103–115

2. Hancock J, Mattick K. Tolerance of ambiguity and psychological well-being in medical training: a systematic review. *Med Educ*. 2020;54(2):125–137

3. Gheihman G, Johnson M, Simpkin AL. Twelve tips for thriving in the face of clinical uncertainty. *Med Teach*. 2020; 42(5):493–499

4. Cristancho S, Lingard L, Forbes T, Ott M, Novick R. Putting the puzzle together: the role of 'problem definition' in complex clinical judgement. *Med Educ*. 2017;51(2):207–214

5. Committee on Diagnostic Error in Health Care; Board on Health Care Services; Institute of Medicine; The National Academies of Sciences, Engineering, and Medicine. In: Balogh EP, ed. *Improving Diagnosis in Health Care*. Washington, DC: National Academies Press; 2015

6. Mamede S, Schmidt HG, Rikers R. Diagnostic errors and reflective practice in medicine. *J Eval Clin Pract*. 2007;13(1):138–145

7. Ilgen JS, Eva KW, de Bruin A, Cook DA, Regehr G. Comfort with uncertainty: reframing our conceptions of how clinicians navigate complex clinical situations. *Adv Health Sci Educ Theory Pract*. 2019;24(4):797–809

8. Crehan E, Scott A. Balint groups as a proposed support mechanism to reduce uncertainty in medical students. *Med Educ*. 2020;54(6):582

9. Hicks PJ, Englander R, Schumacher DJ, et al. Pediatrics milestone project: next steps toward meaningful outcomes assessment. *J Grad Med Educ*. 2010; 2(4):577–584

10. Luther VP, Crandall SJ. Commentary: ambiguity and uncertainty: neglected elements of medical education curricula? *Acad Med*. 2011;86(7): 799–800

11. Beck JB, McGrath C, Toncray K, Rooholamini SN. Failure is an option: using errors as teaching opportunities. *Pediatrics*. 2018;141(3):e20174222

12. Dweck CS. *Mindset: The New Psychology of Success*. New York, NY: Random House; 2006

13. Santhosh L, Chou CL, Connor DM. Diagnostic uncertainty: from education to communication. *Diagnosis (Berl)*. 2019;6(2):121–126

14. Neher JO, Gordon KC, Meyer B, Stevens N. A five-step "microskills" model of clinical teaching. *J Am Board Fam Pract*. 1992;5(4):419–424

15. Arborelius E, Bremberg S, Timpka T. What is going on when the general practitioner doesn't grasp the situation? *Fam Pract*. 1991;8(1):3–9

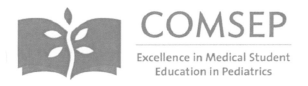

CONTRIBUTORS: Lavjay Butani, MD,[a] Rebecca Blankenburg, MD, MPH,[b] and Michele Long, MD[c]

[a]Department of Pediatrics, University of California Davis Medical Center, Sacramento, California; [b]Stanford University School of Medicine, Stanford, California; and [c]University of California San Francisco, San Francisco, California

Address correspondence to Lavjay Butani, MD, Department of Pediatrics, University of California Davis Medical Center, Ticon 2, Room 348, 2516 Stockton Blvd, Sacramento, CA 95817. E-mail: lbutani@ucdavis.edu

Accepted for publication Nov 12, 2012

doi:10.1542/peds.2012-3106

Stimulating Reflective Practice Among Your Learners

"There are three methods to gaining wisdom. The first is reflection, which is the highest. The second is imitation, which is the easiest. The third is experience, which is the bitterest."

Confucius

Educational organizations, including the Council on Medical Student Education in Pediatrics, recognize that the development of the reflective practitioner is a fundamental element of professional training. The Royal College of Physicians and Surgeons of Canada articulate in their CanMEDS competency framework that physicians must "demonstrate a lifelong commitment to reflective learning" and "recognize and reflect learning issues in practice."[1] Similarly, the Accreditation Council for Graduate Medical Education requires graduating residents to continuously improve patient care based on constant self-evaluation and life-long learning.[2] As part of the ongoing Council on Medical Student Education in Pediatrics series on skills and strategies used by great clinical teachers, this article focuses on reflection, a skill that should be modeled and taught to medical students so that they may practice and refine a reflective approach throughout their careers.

WHAT IS REFLECTION?

Reflection means to "turn back" or think back on experiences. The definition takes on an added meaning when applied to clinical experiences and refers to the process of "slowing down" (not physically, but at an emotional or cognitive level) to analyze, in a deliberate manner, surprising or disconcerting events to make sense of them and understand why they occurred.[3] Critical reflection occurs when one not only explores one's own beliefs, biases, and approaches but also those of others who may have contributed to the way events unfolded. This may lead to a different understanding of what occurred.[3,4] Critical reflection has the potential to promote transformative learning: learning that can be applied to similar, but not necessarily identical, situations that arise in the future.[3,5] The key elements of critical reflection are that it arises out of experience and results in change.

HERE'S ONE WAY TO THINK ABOUT IT

Within medical education, reflection can be categorized into 3 domains: "doctor as expert" (clinical reasoning), "doctor as scholar" (scientific reflection), and "doctor as person" (personal reflection).[6] Within each of these domains, reflection can occur "in action"[7] (like a surgeon analyzing an unexpected problem during surgery by asking, "What am I doing wrong?" or "Why are things not going the way I expected them to?") or "on action"[7] (such as a surgical team debriefing after surgery by asking, "What did we do well, what did we do wrong, and why?"). Ideally, educational strategies should focus on both "in action" and "on action" aspects of reflective practice because they involve different skill sets.

HERE'S HOW TO TEACH REFLECTIVE PRACTICE

While in clinic, a student erroneously diagnoses a febrile 18-month-old child with rhinorrhea, cough, and diffuse symmetric expiratory wheezing as having bacterial pneumonia instead of bronchiolitis. He recommends levofloxacin, based on published adult pneumonia treatment guidelines, and shares that the family was "difficult." His preceptor in this busy clinical environment might be inclined to "help" the student by asking him to read about pneumonia and bronchiolitis, advising him to rely on pediatric literature, and explaining that having a sick child is a very stressful event for a family. Alternatively, this encounter could provide an opportunity to employ a variety of different teaching techniques to promote deeper learning by stimulating reflection, as outlined in the following paragraphs.

Doctor as Expert

"Doctor as an expert" reflection refers to clinical reasoning. For our student, a strategy to promote "reflection in action" could be to ask him to think of an additional diagnosis for this patient besides pneumonia and reprioritize the differential based on the defining and discriminating features of the case[8] (pointing out that the symmetric and diffuse wheezing is atypical for a child with bacterial pneumonia, who is more likely to have focal rhonchi). A "reflection on action" intervention could involve the student using a tool (such as SNAPPS[9] or IDEA[10]) aimed at promoting a structured and systematic clinical reasoning process that encourages the student to defend diagnoses based on key features in the patient's history and physical examination.

Doctor as Scholar

"Doctor as a scholar" reflection involves analyzing and applying evidence-based medicine in patient care encounters. Great teachers encourage learners to pause and reflect on what needs to be considered when applying published literature to their patients. A strategy to promote "reflection in action" could be to lead our student through the exercise of asking PICO (Population, Intervention, Comparison, Outcome)[11] questions as they pertain to this patient because the population addressed in the article he quoted was distinctly different from the patient he saw. The student would then recognize that the findings of the article he chose do not apply to this patient (even if his diagnosis of pneumonia had been correct), stimulating him to learn about differences in etiology and management of pneumonia in different age groups.

A "reflection on action" intervention could involve helping him reflect on an evidence-based practice prescription.[12] After guiding him in framing an appropriate clinical question (such as,

"Compared with adults, what is the most appropriate antibiotic for children with community-acquired pneumonia?"), the student could review the medical literature, choose the most appropriate studies, justify his choices based on an appraisal of the articles, and articulate the application of his findings to improve his patient's care.

Doctor as Person

Reflection on the role of "doctor as a person" attempts to enhance learner empathy by focusing attention on unexplored perspectives of various stakeholders to facilitate emotional engagement. Reflective conversations with medical students can promote professional formation of learners by helping them recommit to humanistic values in the face of common contextual challenges.

For our student, a "reflection in action" strategy could be to have him reflect on, and then verbally present, an account of the events that transpired during his interaction with the family, narrating the events from the perspective of the family, and having him explore how his own beliefs might have

TABLE 1 Strategies to Promote Learning in Each Domain of Reflective Practice

	Sample Strategies for Reflection in Action	Sample Strategies for Reflection on Action
Doctor as a person	Preceptor role modeling of self-awareness and vulnerability.	Appreciative inquiry[13]
	Priming learners to focus on emotions and nonverbal cues in patient interactions.	Narrative writing[14]
	Skill-building exercises focused on improving "mindfulness," cultivating "engaged curiosity," and improving observation of events such as perspective-taking and role-playing workshops.[19]	Reflections on critical incident reports, formative events, and multisource feedback.[20] Role modeling of reflection
Doctor as an expert	Diagnostic "pauses," with focus on justifying the differential diagnosis based on discriminating features of illnesses.	Horizontal reading[8]
	One-Minute-Preceptor[21]	IDEA[10]: • Interpretive summary • Differential diagnosis with commitment to the most likely diagnosis • Explanation of reasoning in choosing the most likely diagnosis • Alternative diagnoses with explanation of reasoning SNAPPS[9]: • Summarize history and findings; narrow the differential • Analyze the differential • Probe preceptor • Plan management • Select issue for self-directed learning
Doctor as a scholar	Debriefing on errors/near-errors based on inappropriate application of literature in clinical decision-making.	Evidence-based practice prescriptions[12]
	PICO[11]: • Population • Intervention • Comparison • Outcome	5 A's of evidence-based practice[22]: • Ask • Acquire • Appraise • Apply • Analyze

impacted the interaction. One could then have the learner re-engage the family to address their concerns and beliefs pertaining to their child's respiratory illness. Even such brief oral reflective exercises have a profound impact, because they occur in close relation to the event and may positively influence the outcome. A "reflection on action" strategy could involve the learner writing a reflective paragraph describing multiple perspectives such as his own, the family's, the preceptor's, and even that of the education literature (as it pertains to difficult patient interactions). Alternatively, the student could interview a mentor of his choice to learn how the mentor has successfully addressed similar difficult encounters with patients and reflect on the experience (appreciative inquiry).[13]

CHALLENGES TO PROMOTING REFLECTION

Challenges exist for both the learner and the preceptor. Learner reflective capacity can be quite variable,[14] and students may be apprehensive to critically reflect, as sensitive issues may be discussed. Preceptors may feel pressed for time or not aware of how to promote reflection. Table 1 lists techniques that can be used to promote learning in each of the domains of reflection.

CONCLUSIONS

Medicine is full of conundrums and challenges, both cognitive and emotional. Reflective habits assist practitioners in addressing and managing unexpected situations and challenges for which there is no one right answer and enable them to learn and grow from these experiences.[15] Although there is admittedly limited evidence

specifically supporting a link between reflective teaching interventions and patient care outcomes, a growing body of medical education literature is accumulating, demonstrating that reflective learning promotes professional formation,[16] empathy,[17] and clinical reasoning skills.[18]

ACKNOWLEDGMENTS
The authors acknowledge Drs Janice Hanson, Christopher Maloney, and Susan Bannister for their thoughtful review and editing of the article.

REFERENCES

1. The CanMEDS 2005 physician competency framework. In: Frank J, ed. *Better Standards. Better Physicians. Better Care.* Ottawa, Ontario, Canada: The Royal College of Physicians and Surgeons of Canada; 2005

2. Swing SR. The ACGME outcome project: retrospective and prospective. *Med Teach.* 2007; 29(7):648–654

3. Mezirow J. How critical reflection triggers transformative learning. In: Mezirow JA, ed. *Fostering Critical Reflection in Adulthood: A Guide to Transformative and Emancipatory Learning.* San Francisco, CA: Jossey-Bass; 1990:1–6

4. Aronson L. Twelve tips for teaching reflection at all levels of medical education. *Med Teach.* 2011;33(3):200–205

5. Aronson L, Niehaus B, Hill-Sakurai L, Lai C, O'Sullivan PS. A comparison of two methods of teaching reflective ability in Year 3 medical students. *Med Educ.* 2012;46(8):807–814

6. Aukes LC, Geertsma J, Cohen-Schotanus J, Zwierstra RP, Slaets JP. The development of a scale to measure personal reflection in medical practice and education. *Med Teach.* 2007;29(2-3):177–182

7. Schon DA. *The Reflective Practitioner: How Professionals Think in Action.* New York, NY: Basic Books; 1984

8. Bowen JL. Educational strategies to promote clinical diagnostic reasoning. *N Engl J Med.* 2006;355(21):2217–2225

9. Wolpaw TM, Wolpaw DR, Papp KK. SNAPPS: a learner-centered model for outpatient

education. *Acad Med.* 2003;78(9):893–898

10. Baker ELC, Liston B. Teaching, evaluating, and remediating clinical reasoning. *Academic Internal Medicine Insight.* 2010;8(1): 12–13

11. Richardson WS, Wilson MC, Nishikawa J, Hayward RS. The well-built clinical question: a key to evidence-based decisions. *ACP J Club.* 1995;123(3):A12–A13

12. Rucker L, Morrison E. The "EBM Rx": an initial experience with an evidence-based learning prescription. *Acad Med.* 2000;75 (5):527–528

13. Quaintance JL, Arnold L, Thompson GS. What students learn about professionalism from faculty stories: an "appreciative inquiry" approach. *Acad Med.* 2010;85(1): 118–123

14. DasGupta S, Charon R. Personal illness narratives: using reflective writing to teach empathy. *Acad Med.* 2004;79(4):351–356

15. Sandars J. The use of reflection in medical education: AMEE Guide No. 44. *Med Teach.* 2009;31(8):685–695

16. Stark P, Roberts C, Newble D, Bax N. Discovering professionalism through guided reflection. *Med Teach.* 2006;28(1):e25–e31

17. Misra-Hebert AD, Issacson JH, Kohn M, et al. Improving empathy of physicians through guided reflective writing. *Int J Med Educ.* 2012;3:71–77

18. Mamede S, van Gog T, Moura AS, et al. Reflection as a strategy to foster medical students' acquisition of diagnostic competence. *Med Educ.* 2012;46(5):464–472

19. Halpern J. Empathy and patient-physician conflicts. *J Gen Intern Med.* 2007;22(5): 696–700

20. Sargeant JM, Mann KV, van der Vleuten CP, Metsemakers JF. Reflection: a link between receiving and using assessment feedback. *Adv Health Sci Educ Theory Pract.* 2009;14 (3):399–410

21. Furney SL, Orsini AN, Orsetti KE, Stern DT, Gruppen LD, Irby DM. Teaching the one-minute preceptor. A randomized controlled trial. *J Gen Intern Med.* 2001;16(9): 620–624

22. Green ML. Evaluating evidence-based practice. In: Holmboe ES, Hawkins RE, eds. *Practical Guide to the Evaluation of Clinical Competence.* 1st ed. Philadelphia, PA: Mosby, Inc.; 2008:130–148

FINANCIAL DISCLOSURE: *The authors have indicated they have no financial relationships relevant to this article to disclose.*
FUNDING: No external funding.

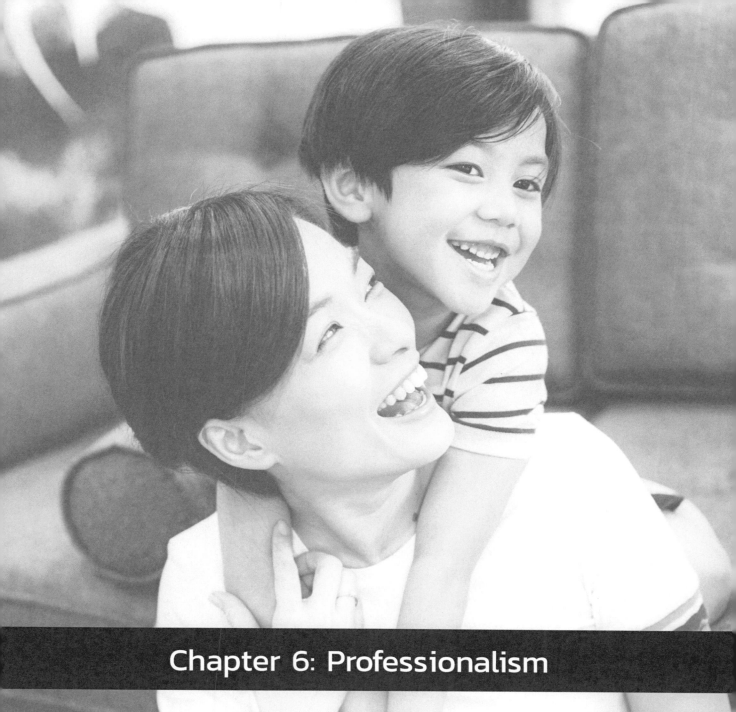

Chapter 6: Professionalism

Chapter 6

Fostering Professionalism Among the Next Generation of Medical Professionals

By Terry Kind, MD, MPH
Professor of Pediatrics, The George Washington University School of Medicine and Health Sciences

The charge of medical education is lofty: to train the next generation of healthcare professionals. In order to earn and maintain the public's trust, medical knowledge, skills, behaviors, and attitudes must be anchored in a foundation of professionalism. Across the continuum from student to physician there is a responsibility to patients, families, and communities. This applies to those who are forming their professional identities and to those who are treating patients and teaching others. This applies across all communities, including those where there are health inequities and injustices to remedy. Teaching about social determinants of health and embracing work on diversity, equity, and inclusion in medical schools is a key component of today's professionalism for tomorrow's health professionals.

Professionalism in pediatrics is framed as something to *strive* for, as the "ideal standards of behavior and professional practice to which pediatricians should aspire and by which students and residents can be evaluated."[1] Professionalism is part of being or becoming a "good doctor." This comprehensive concept includes honesty and integrity, reliability and responsibility, respect for others, compassion and empathy, and effective communication and collaboration. It also means having an awareness of one's own limits and working to improve oneself, while advocating for and serving others.[2]

Notably, it has been established that unprofessional behavior in medical school, such as irresponsibility and a diminished capacity for self-improvement, is associated with subsequent disciplinary action by a medical board.[3] This landmark case-control study by Papadakis et al[3] provided evidence that physicians disciplined by state licensing boards were much more likely to have demonstrated unprofessional behaviors as medical students than matched controls. Among various other potential factors, lack of professionalism as a student was the strongest predictor of disciplinary action. Consider the impact if those medical student unprofessional behaviors had been identified and remediated. Medical educators must teach, assess, and promote professionalism and address lapses among learners. Recognizing how critical it is to teach and assess professionalism, there are accreditation standards requiring that medical schools ensure that learning environments are conducive to the ongoing development of professional behaviors.[4] Accordingly, medical schools must develop strategies to enhance positive and mitigate negative influences and promptly correct violations of professional standards.

There are 3 articles in this chapter that address professionalism in a range of important ways.

In "Professionalism in Practice: Strategies for Assessment, Remediation, and Promotion," several useful tools are elucidated.[5] Just as assessing the learner's knowledge and skills are part of everyday clinical education, it is also the responsibility of every clinical teacher to assess a learner's professionalism. Identifying and remediating lapses early is critical to the learner's development. Some observable and assessable components of professionalism are the student's adherence to ethical principles, their effective interactions with teammates and patients, their reliability and accountability, and their commitment to improvement.

Lapses in professionalism can take the form of behaviors, performance, attitudes, or lack of accountability, and using these categorizations can help in discussing with the student and planning remediation strategies. Particularly helpful in this article are key statements that clinical educators can use when discussing lapses with learners. This includes conveying that one of the physician's roles is to assist the learner in their professional growth and development, and to let the learner know how their behaviors were perceived.

The next article in this chapter turns to millennial learners. "Supporting the Development of Professional Identity in the Millennial Leaner" is based on the premise that building an identity as a physician is the foundation for professional behaviors.[6] For clinical educators with concerns about the preparedness of millennials (born 1981–2000) to meet the profession's expectations, this piece provides a framework to assist with learners' professional identity formation. Drawing on autonomy, competence and relatedness of self-determination theory, the framework's acronym is I-CA^{2}R^{2}E. Here, clinical teachers make individual connections, they create (safe spaces and opportunities), they acknowledge what's going on and adjust their views, they reflect (and encourage reflection), they role model, and they have an exchange with the millennial learner. Three case scenarios provide the clinical educator with solutions for the potential issues of the performance-focused learner, the self-interested learner with misplaced priorities, and the learner with a limited viewpoint.

The third article in this series draws upon all the above principles and helps the clinical educator interested in "Opting in to Online Professionalism: Social Media and Pediatrics."[7] This piece encourages pediatric educators to have a social media action plan and provides guiding questions that facilitate reflection on one's own social media identity and an exploration of goals, actions, interactions, and opportunities online. There are noted caveats as well as ways to actively promote professionalism among students. First and foremost is maintaining patient privacy, as well as maintaining appropriate boundaries just as one would in other contexts. Then comes knowing and monitoring one's online presence and recognizing the impact one's actions can have on the public trust, whether negatively or positively. Professionalism lapses online loom large due to ease of dissemination and amplification. With a positive presence on social media, physician educators can add value by modeling professionalism, providing accurate information, countering inaccuracies, advocating to address health inequities, and connecting with others in health care for teaching and learning.

These perspectives remind us that it is the clinical educator's responsibility to model professionalism in both the familiar and in new settings, to assess and remediate professionalism among trainees and foster their professional identity formation, and to uphold the physician's contract with society.

References:
1. Fallat ME, Glover J, and the Committee on Bioethics. Professionalism in Pediatrics. *Pediatrics*. 2007;120;e1123.
2. ABMS Professionalism Work Group. Definitions of Medical Professionalism (Long Form). 2012 Available at: https://www.abms.org/media/84742/abms-definition-of-medical-professionalism.pdf. Accessed October 26, 2020.
3. Papadakis MA, Teherani A, Banach MA et al. Disciplinary Action by Medical Boards and Prior Behavior in Medical School. *N Engl J Med*. 2005;353:2673-82.
4. Liaison Committee on Medical Education. Functions and Structure of a Medical School: Standards for Accreditation of Medical Education Programs Leading to the MD Degree. March 2020. Available at: https://lcme.org/publications. Accessed October 26, 2020
5. Buchanan AO, Stallworth J, Christy C, Garfunkel LC, Hanson JL. Professionalism in practice: strategies for assessment, remediation, and promotion. *Pediatrics*. 2012;129(3):407-9.
6. Barone MA, Vercio C, Jirasevijinda T. Supporting the Development of Professional Identity in the Millennial Learner. *Pediatrics*. 2019;143(3):e20183988.
7. Kind T, Patel PD, Lie DA. Opting in to online professionalism: social media and pediatrics. *Pediatrics*. 2013;132(5):792-5.

PEDIATRICS PERSPECTIVES

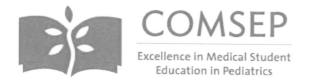

Excellence in Medical Student
Education in Pediatrics

CONTRIBUTORS: April O. Buchanan, MD,[a] James Stallworth, MD,[b] Cynthia Christy, MD,[c] Lynn C. Garfunkel, MD,[c] and Janice L. Hanson, PhD, EdS[d]

[a]Department of Pediatrics, University of South Carolina School of Medicine, Greenville Hospital System University Medical Center, Greenville, South Carolina; [b]Division of General Pediatrics, Department of Pediatrics, University of South Carolina School of Medicine, Columbia, South Carolina; [c]Department of Pediatrics, University of Rochester School of Medicine, Rochester General Hospital, Rochester, New York; and [d]Department of Pediatrics, University of Colorado School of Medicine, The Children's Hospital, Medical Education, Aurora, Colorado

Address correspondence to April O. Buchanan, MD, Department of Pediatrics, University of South Carolina School of Medicine, Greenville Hospital System University Medical Center, 701 Grove Rd, 4th Floor Balcony Suites, Greenville, SC 29605. E-mail: abuchanan@ghs.org

Accepted for publication Dec 21, 2011

doi:10.1542/peds.2011-3716

Professionalism in Practice: Strategies for Assessment, Remediation, and Promotion

The Council on Medical Student Education in Pediatrics continues its series on great clinical teachers, focusing on professionalism in practice. The Council on Medical Student Education in Pediatrics is in agreement with the Liaison Committee on Medical Education, Accreditation Council on Graduate Medical Education, and the CanMEDS Physician Competency Framework, that professionalism is essential to the practice of medicine, regardless of the level of training. Clinical teachers are in an excellent position to promote and assess professional behaviors in students but are often hesitant to address lapses in professionalism; however, addressing professionalism early is critical, as professional misbehavior in medical school is a major risk factor for subsequent censure by state medical boards.[1] This article discusses tools and strategies for the assessment, remediation, and promotion of professionalism in medical students.

Professionalism in Practice

Many practitioners say, "I know it when I see it," but defining professionalism can be challenging. Professionalism is built on the principles of excellence, humanism, accountability, and altruism and is demonstrated through clinical competence, communication, and ethical understanding.[2] Humanism and altruism encompass beneficence, respect, truthfulness, and placing the needs of the patient above one's own. Excellence and accountability include striving for high-quality patient care, making a commitment to lifelong learning, and exhibiting responsibility to duty. Professional maturity requires the development of these behaviors through deliberate practice so that they become the habits that define a good physician. Evaluating professionalism is the responsibility of every clinical teacher. Assessable components include adherence to ethical practice principles,

effective interactions with patients and the people who are important to these patients, effective interactions with individuals within the health care system, reliability and accountability, and commitment to improvement.[3]

Tools for Assessment

The development of professionalism in medical students takes place under a wide variety of conditions in all years of medical school. Assessment, therefore, must take place over time and in authentic settings, highlighting the importance of clinical teachers in assessing student professionalism. Specific observations provide the most accurate evaluations, and multiple observations and observers help ensure reliability and validity.[4] Instruments for assessing professionalism include faculty narratives and rating tools, multirater evaluations, reflective writing, and reports of unprofessional behavior.

Many clinical teachers are familiar with rating scales that list criteria and descriptors to determine where students fall on a continuum for a variety of competencies and usually include space for a narrative. Several rating scales have been developed that specifically evaluate attributes of professionalism.[5,6] Advantages of rating scales include familiarity, ease of distribution, and opportunity for commentary. A major disadvantage is limited reliability, especially when teachers are not trained in the use of a specific instrument.

Multirater evaluations often provide a more comprehensive picture of student performance and insight into otherwise hard-to-evaluate behaviors. Instruments, such as the Musick 360-degree,[7] can be completed by physicians, nurses, and other health care personnel, whereas tools, such as the Wake Forest Physician Trust Scheme,[8] are completed by patients and caregivers. Although these tools can provide feedback to learners on a wide range of behaviors and actions, their use can be time and labor intensive, and results may be affected by patient/parent literacy, language, culture, and personality. Regardless of the tool used, the instrument should focus on behaviors rather than personal characteristics. Clinical teachers will need to clearly define to whom the instruments will be distributed and how they will be collected.

Reflective writing is the process by which a student reflects on the meaning or impact of a specific observed incident or case-based scenario.[9] Reflective writing allows for purposeful contemplation and lends itself to feedback. Scales to analyze the level of student reflection and understanding have been developed.[10] Reflective writing is time-consuming for both teachers and students, and teachers often need additional training to feel comfortable with this approach. Nevertheless, reserving time to discuss the student's written feelings and insight can help foster a meaningful student-physician relationship and encourage professional growth.

Finally, some schools use incident reports to document and track unprofessional behaviors by medical students.[11] For each professional lapse, the preceptor completes a standardized form describing the context and nature of the lapse. The incident reports are stored centrally and periodically reviewed by a committee, with possible referral to a promotions or standards committee, depending on the severity or the repetitiveness of the lapses. Effective use of these reports requires a shared vocabulary and understanding of the definition of professionalism among students and faculty. Quick access to the forms, a seamless method of submission, and clear policies regarding management of the report are required for successful implementation.

Strategies for Remediation

A lapse in professionalism should be categorized as behavior (eg, lack of respect for patients), performance (eg, inability to concentrate on tasks at hand), attitude (eg, lack of humility or overconfidence), or lack of accountability (eg, frequent tardiness). Categorizing the lapse will help when discussing the lapse with the student and determining the best course for a remediation plan. Specific information about the context of the incident should be included in the documentation of the professional lapse.[12] Although the clinical teacher can address issues, such as dress codes, punctuality, communication, and attention to studies, issues related to the student's mental health or impaired performance secondary to substance use should be referred to the dean's office. Many medical schools have multidisciplinary committees that help in dealing with students with professional issues, so knowing the resources available is useful.

Successful remediation requires an organized approach to the student's professional lapse. Steps include the following: (1) confirm the lapse, (2) understand the context, (3) communicate and discuss in a mutually respectful manner, (4) encourage self-reflection, (5) agree on a plan for remediation, (6) document the interventions, and (7) construct a plan for follow-up.[13] Table 1 lists some strategies for communication with the student; these are useful especially when a lapse is reported secondhand. Each type of professional transgression requires a different approach and individualized remediation plan. The plan should be written and include the characterization of lapse, goal(s), requirements for reading, specific behavioral change goal(s), a plan for monitoring or reassessing, and consequences for relapse.[13,14] More than 1 discussion may be needed so the student has time to reflect on the professional lapse and the initial conversation.

A student's response to clear communication from the teacher gives insight into the student's conscientiousness, an aspect of professionalism for which an

TABLE 1 Statements for Communication When Discussing Lapses in Professionalism[14]

"You don't have to agree with me, but I want you to understand me."

"I am not saying you are totally at fault but we need to work together to help you understand what is viewed as a professional lapse."

"I realize this is tough to talk about, but my job is to help make you be the best physician possible."

"If you were on this side of the desk, how would you handle this issue?"

"I understand there may be disagreement about this issue, but I need to let you know the way you are being perceived."

"You may have meant it in another way, but you were perceived as being unprofessional."

index has been developed.[15] Responses, such as remorse or apology, rather than anger or denial, and accepting responsibility for the lapse improve the odds that the lapse is remediable.

Barriers to Remediating Lapses in Professionalism

Barriers to remediating lapses in professionalism include inappropriate or paucity of tools, the time necessary to intervene, worry over future impact to the student's career, professed lack of skills to address the issues, the potential for impaired relationships, and fear of student retribution or litigation.[4] Clear communication with the clerkship director and delineation of responsibilities can help alleviate some of these concerns.

Promoting Professionalism

Clinical teachers play an important role in supporting the development of professional behaviors among medical students by modeling professionalism in their own day-to-day interactions with patients, families, staff, and learners.[16] If a patient, nurse, or staff member compliments the student on a professional behavior, the clinical teacher should make sure the behavior is acknowledged. Possible ways include directly praising the student, specifically listing the comment on the student evaluation tool, sending an e-mail to the clerkship director, or completing a praise card for exemplary behavior,[17] if available. For those students who continue to demonstrate exemplary behavior throughout medical school, providing an award as recognition may help affirm the importance of professionalism to the institution.

Summary

Great clinical teachers promote professional behavior and, although challenging, identify and correct professional lapses in students. Several tools and strategies exist to help clinical teachers assess and remediate professionalism in medical students. Although many lapses in professionalism by students can be effectively managed by the faculty preceptor, some incidents may require discussion with the clerkship director or other representatives from the medical school. Helping medical students develop habits of excellence, humanism, accountability, and altruism is one our great professional responsibilities and is rewarded by the continued trust of patients in their physicians.

ACKNOWLEDGMENTS

We thank our editors, Christopher Maloney, Alexandra Clark, and William Raszka, for their helpful comments and thoughtful reviews of the manuscript.

REFERENCES

1. Papadakis MA, Teherani A, Banach MA, et al. Disciplinary action by medical boards and prior behavior in medical school. *N Engl J Med.* 2005;353(25):2673–2682

2. Stern DT, ed. *Measuring Medical Professionalism*. New York, NY: Oxford University Press; 2006

3. Wilkinson TJ, Wade WB, Knock LD. A blueprint to assess professionalism: results of a systematic review. *Acad Med.* 2009;84(5): 551–558

4. Thistlethwaite J, Spencer J. *Professionalism in Medicine*. Abingdon, UK: Radcliffe Publishing; 2008

5. Gauger PG, Gruppen LD, Minter RM, Colletti LM, Stern DT. Initial use of a novel instrument to measure professionalism in surgical residents. *Am J Surg.* 2005;189(4): 479–487

6. van de Camp K, Vernooij-Dassen MJ, Grol RP, Bottema BJ. Professionalism in general practice: development of an instrument to assess professional behaviour in general practitioner trainees. *Med Educ.* 2006;40 (1):43–50

7. Musick DW, McDowell SM, Clark N, Salcido R. Pilot study of a 360-degree assessment instrument for physical medicine & rehabilitation residency programs. *Am J Phys Med Rehabil.* 2003;82(5):394–402

8. Hall MA, Zheng B, Dugan E, et al. Measuring patients' trust in their primary care providers. *Med Care Res Rev.* 2002;59(3):293–318

9. Stark P, Roberts C, Newble D, Bax N. Discovering professionalism through guided reflection. *Med Teach.* 2006;28(1):e25–e31

10. Aukes LC, Geertsma J, Cohen-Schotanus J, Zwierstra RP, Slaets JPJ. The development of a scale to measure personal reflection in medical practice and education. *Med Teach.* 2007;29(2-3):177–182

11. Papadakis MA, Loeser H, Healy K. Early detection and evaluation of professionalism deficiencies in medical students: one school's approach. *Acad Med.* 2001;76(11): 1100–1106

12. Ginsburg S, Regehr G, Hatala R, et al. Context, conflict, and resolution: a new conceptual framework for evaluating professionalism. *Acad Med.* 2000;75(suppl 10):S6–S11

13. Trimm F, Bar-on M. Preparing remediation plans: are you the next design star? (workshop). Pediatric Academic Societies, Baltimore, MD. May 2, 2009

14. Christy C, Garfunkel L, Stallworth J. Remediating unprofessional behavior across the continuum (workshop). Pediatric Academic Societies, Vancouver. May 2, 2010

15. McLachlan JC, Finn G, Macnaughton J. The conscientiousness index: a novel tool to explore students' professionalism. *Acad Med.* 2009;84(5):559–565

16. Brownell AKW, Côté L. Senior residents' views on the meaning of professionalism and how they learn about it. *Acad Med.* 2001;76(7):734–737

17. University of Illinois Chicago. Professionalism evaluation form for medical students. Available at: https://www.uic.edu/ com/dom/gim/ambcourse/Prof-Form.doc. Accessed December 9, 2011

FINANCIAL DISCLOSURE: *The authors have indicated they have no financial relationships relevant to this article to disclose.*
FUNDING: No external funding.

Supporting the Development of Professional Identity in the Millennial Learner

Michael A. Barone, MD, MPH,[a,b] Chad Vercio, MD,[c,d] Thanakorn Jirasevijinda, MD[e]

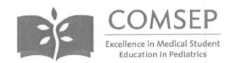

As teachers, we train learners to be knowledgeable and competent in the practice of medicine. No less important is the way teachers impact the development of learners' professional identity. Social scientists in the 1950s noted medical education's charge "to shape the novice into the effective practitioner of medicine, to give [them] the best available knowledge and skills, and to provide [the novice] with a professional identity so that [they] come to think, act, and feel like a physician."[1] Many have stressed the importance of curricula focused on learners' personal and professional development.[2] An awareness of professional identity development helps teachers understand some of the workplace differences noted between generations, particularly with millennial learners.

Continuing the Council on Medical Student Education in Pediatrics series on great clinical teachers, our article focuses on supporting professional identity formation (PIF) in millennial learners.

Professional identity formation (ie, the socialization and professionalization of a physician) develops in stages over time.[3] PIF consists of ordering and reordering personal and professional priorities as one progresses from student to effective practitioner.[3–5] This process has been linked to one's personal identity development.[6] Characteristics of 3 important stages of physician PIF include the following[5]:

Early: foundational education (premedical students and early medical students)

- follow social roles and rules
- appreciate others' viewpoints, yet self-views predominate;

Middle: training and/or supervised practice (later medical students and residents)

- view medical practice through multiple perspectives
- subordinate self-interests more effectively
- feel a sense of belonging but not yet "professional"
- may still have trouble reconciling competing expectations;

Later: practicing professional (practicing physicians)

- understand differing values and perspectives
- own and embody expectations of the profession
- begin to internalize the external values of the profession
- reconcile challenges between personal and professional expectations more effectively.

An identity as a physician is the foundation for professional behaviors. For example, a major pillar of professionalism is a commitment to maintaining trust by subordinating self-interest and

[a]National Board of Medical Examiners, Philadelphia, Pennsylvania; [b]School of Medicine, Johns Hopkins University, Baltimore, Maryland; [c]School of Medicine, Loma Linda University, Loma Linda, California; [d]Riverside University Health System, Moreno Valley, California; and [e]Weill Cornell Medical College, Cornell University, New York, New York

Drs Barone, Vercio, and Jirasevijinda conceptualized and drafted the initial manuscript and reviewed and revised the manuscript; and all authors approved the final manuscript as submitted and agree to be accountable for all aspects of the work.

DOI: https://doi.org/10.1542/peds.2018-3988

Accepted for publication Dec 17, 2018

Address correspondence to Michael A. Barone, MD, MPH, National Board of Medical Examiners, 3750 Market St, Philadelphia, PA 19104. E-mail: mbarone@nbme.org

PEDIATRICS (ISSN Numbers: Print, 0031-4005; Online, 1098-4275).

FINANCIAL DISCLOSURE: The authors have indicated they have no financial relationships relevant to this article to disclose.

FUNDING: No external funding.

POTENTIAL CONFLICT OF INTEREST: The authors have indicated they have no potential conflicts of interest to disclose.

To cite: Barone MA, Vercio C, Jirasevijinda T. Supporting the Development of Professional Identity in the Millennial Learner. *Pediatrics.* 2019;143(3):e20183988

managing professional responsibilities.[5,7] Through acknowledgment, questioning, and role modeling, clinical teachers can support a learner's professional identity development, ensuring smooth transitions. Understanding personal identity formation and PIF is central to teaching, mentoring, and remediating learners.

Concern exists about the millennial generation's preparedness to meet the expectations of the profession. Millennials (born 1981–2000) are said to have been reared in a "child-focused" world with high parental involvement and relationships shaped by media.[8] In medicine, millennials have been characterized as having less commitment to and ownership of patients, a work life shaped more by personal demands, and a sense of greater importance to an organization despite a relative lack of experience. These factors could lead to conflicts with teachers about expectations and commitment.[9,10] Nonetheless, millennials bring many strengths to medicine, such as collaborative learning, acceptance of diversity, and a strong sense of social consciousness.[11] In Table 1, we summarize millennials' characteristics that potentially impact PIF in positive and negative ways.

Generational differences between teachers and learners may create conflicts. We propose the I-CA^{2}R^{2}E (individual connection, create, acknowledge and adjust, reflect and role model, and exchange) framework (Table 1) to provide strategies to maximize learners' PIF. The framework addresses the 3 pillars of Self-Determination Theory, which are autonomy, competence, and relatedness.[12] The 3 brief cases that follow illustrate how I-CA^{2}R^{2}E can help guide clinical teachers.

CASE 1: THE PERFORMANCE-FOCUSED LEARNER

A clerkship student meets with her preceptor to discuss dissatisfaction with feedback she received, concerned that the preceptor pointed out areas for improvement.

Potential Issues

The learner, in her early stage of PIF, may view clinical work in a self-focused manner and perceive feedback as judgment and not an opportunity for growth.[11]

Proposed Solutions Using the I-CA^{2}R^{2}E Framework

I - Make individual connection and explore the learner's experience with previous feedback.

C - Create a safe space to discuss how the feedback impacts the learner's view of herself and her role (ie, as test taker versus lifelong learner).

A - Acknowledge grading pressures in medical school and the learner's concerns that grades are "all that matters" for residency selection.

A - Adjust your own views on feedback and recognize how generational differences play a role in how feedback is received.

R - Reflect: encourage reflection on key influences in the learner's identity development (mentors, patients, other experiences).

R - Role model by sharing how feedback has benefitted you (for example, how listening to the observations and perspectives of others provided opportunities for personal and professional growth).

E - Exchange: arrange for follow-up with the learner to check in on challenges and successes.

CASE 2: THE SELF-INTERESTED LEARNER WITH MISPLACED PRIORITIES

A subintern visiting from another institution is upset because of his attending's raising concerns about his level of commitment. The subintern's assignment on his patient's adjustment to a serious diagnosis was submitted late. When asked, the subintern explains he "prefers taking care of his patients" and that written assignments "matter less" than clinical care.

Potential Issues

The learner may not fully be able to subordinate self-interests and have trouble reconciling competing priorities.

Proposed Solutions Using the I-CA^{2}R^{2}E Framework

I - Make a connection by exploring personal background and career goals.

C - Create a safe space to explore how this learner prioritizes competing commitments.

A - Acknowledge that competing demands can be difficult to manage.

A - Adjust your own potential biases about this learner being "dis-engaged" or "uninterested."

R - Reflect: encourage the learner's reflection on his ordering of priorities.

R - Role model by sharing how you have grappled with managing competing priorities.

E - Exchange: provide rationale for assignments and offer to assist and exchange ideas about the how this subintern can order future priorities.

CASE 3: THE LEARNER WITH A LIMITED VIEWPOINT

A senior resident objects to the residency program's decision to limit intern shifts to 16 hours. He complains program leadership is "getting soft" and publicly challenges other residents for having supported the program's decision.

Potential Issues

The learner may have a limited ability to consider multiple perspectives.

TABLE 1 Millennial Attributes That May Positively and Negatively Interact With PIF and the I-CA^{2}R^{2}E Framework

Millennial Attributes Potentially Impacting Physician Identity Development	Methods to Address I-CA^{2}R^{2}E	Comments

Positive interaction
  Relationship centered
  Expect personal connection with supervisors
Negative interaction
  Conflict with hierarchy
  Occasional distrust of authority
	Individual connection	Connect with learners through a variety of methods and determine a preferred method; pay attention to the learner's journey to medicine and outside interests.

Positive interaction
  Equality and diversity
  Team centered and collaborative learning
Negative interaction
  Personal learning needs are valued more than group learning and/or team training
	Create	Create a safe space for honest dialogue; provide opportunities for learners to share the important experiences and pivotal moments in their identity development as a physician (ie, the process of becoming medical professional).

Positive interaction
  Desires routine feedback
  Social consciousness
Negative interaction
  Easily bored with traditional education (didactics)
  May have trouble with independent decision-making
  Frustrated with "menial" tasks
	Acknowledge and adjust	Acknowledge learner perspectives; validate story and concerns; adjust approaches on the basis of learner values, reactions, stage of life, and training; adjust teaching methods on the basis of learner preferences; and adjust and challenge your own expectations of "what is right."

Positive interaction
  Desire for meaning in work
Negative interaction
  May view feedback as judgment and not an opportunity for growth
  Need for explicit instructions
	Reflect and role model	Encourage reflection on personal experiences; provide nonjudgmental feedback when values and ideals conflict; role model expected behavior; and coach as learners order and reorder priorities.

	Exchange	Arrange for ongoing dialogue, connection, and follow-up; if learners acknowledge ongoing problems, ask if they would like to hear potential solutions.

The senior resident's emotional approach to sharing his perspective is not productive.

Proposed Solutions Using the I-CA^{2}R^{2}E Framework

I - Recognize this resident's individual perspective as he approaches unsupervised practice.

C - Create an opportunity for the resident to articulate rationale, not simply emotional reactions.

A - Acknowledge that the resident is entitled to his point of view, yet the decision-making process (program leadership and other resident input) should be respected. Encourage the resident to focus on outcomes and not only resident work hours.

A - Adjust your personal biases and understand that generational differences impact expectations of learners.

R - Reflect and role model: probe the resident's view on how his action manifested as role modeling for others (ie, hours in the hospital versus a focus on quality, safety, and relationships with patients). Reflect on a time when your own first impressions were modified over time.

E - Exchange: set a time for follow-up and ask for ideas about how future group decisions can be collaborative.

CONCLUSIONS

Although it may seem a distant memory to great clinical teachers, the early stages of a medical learner's PIF can be disconcerting and filled with conflict, self-doubt, and an inadequate sense of belonging to the profession. Millennial learners may particularly need guidance through challenges to make critical decisions (ordering and reordering priorities) that ultimately lead to the embodiment of professional behaviors (ie, thinking, acting, and feeling like a physician). Supervisors who approach teachable moments with open-mindedness, a willingness to challenge expectations, and tools to stimulate exploration and self-reflection (I-CA^{2}R^{2}E) will be able to promote learners' development of a strong foundational identity in medicine. When learners experience the investment of a clinical teacher in their professional journey, everyone benefits, including patients, who ultimately receive care from physicians who truly embody the expectations of the medical profession above their own needs.

ACKNOWLEDGMENT

We thank Dr Nicholas Potisek for his thoughtful contributions in conceptualizing this article.

ABBREVIATIONS

I-CA^{2}R^{2}E: individual connection, create, acknowledge and adjust, reflect and role model, and exchange

PIF: professional identity formation

REFERENCES

1. Merton RK, Reader GG, Kendall PL, eds. *The Student-Physician: Introductory Studies in the Sociology of Medical Education.* Cambridge, MA: Published for the Commonwealth Fund by Harvard University Press; 1957

2. Inui TS. *A Flag in the Wind: Educating for Professionalism in Medicine.* Washington, DC: Association of American Medical Colleges; 2003

3. Johnston S. See one, do one, teach one: developing professionalism across the generations. *Clin Orthop Relat Res.* 2006;449(449):186–192

4. Cruess SR, Cruess RL. Teaching professionalism - why, what and how. *Facts Views Vis ObGyn.* 2012;4(4): 259–265

5. Cruess RL, Cruess SR, Boudreau JD, Snell L, Steinert Y. A schematic representation of the professional identity formation and socialization of medical students and residents: a guide for medical educators. *Acad Med.* 2015; 90(6):718–725

6. Kegan R. *The Evolving Self: Problem and Process in Human Development.* Cambridge, MA: Harvard University Press; 1982

7. American Board of Internal Medicine Foundation. The physician charter. Available at: http://abimfoundation.org/what-we-do/physician-charter. Accessed November 1, 2018

8. Clark University. About the Clark University poll. Clark University poll. Available at: http://www2.clarku.edu/clark-poll-emerging-adults/. Accessed November 1, 2018

9. Eckleberry-Hunt J, Tucciarone J. The challenges and opportunities of teaching "generation y". *J Grad Med Educ.* 2011;3(4):458–461

10. Shaw H. *Sticking Points: How to Get 4 Generations Working Together in the 12 Places They Come Apart.* Carol Stream, IL: Tyndale House Publishers; 2013

11. Lancaster LC, Stillman D, Mackay H. *When Generations Collide: Who They Are, Why They Clash, How to Solve the Generational Puzzle at Work.* New York, NY: Collins Business; 2005

12. Kusurkar R, ten Cate O. AM last page: education is not filling a bucket, but lighting a fire: self-determination theory and motivation in medical students. *Acad Med.* 2013;88(6):904

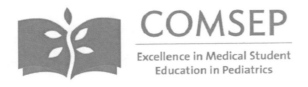

AUTHORS: Terry Kind, MD, MPH,[a] Pradip D. Patel, MD,[b] and Desiree A. Lie, MD, MSED[c]

[a]Department of Pediatrics, Children's National Medical Center, George Washington University, Washington, District of Columbia; [b]Department of Pediatrics, University of Louisville School of Medicine, Louisville, Kentucky; and [c]Department of Family Medicine, Keck School of Medicine of the University of Southern California, Los Angeles, California

Address correspondence to Terry Kind, MD, MPH, Children's National Medical Center, 111 Michigan Ave, NW, Washington, DC 20010. E-mail: tkind@childrensnational.org; @kind4kids (Twitter)

Accepted for publication Aug 7, 2013

KEY WORDS
professionalism, social media

ABBREVIATION
AMA—American Medical Association

Dr Kind conceptualized and designed the feature and drafted the initial manuscript; Drs Patel and Lie reviewed and revised the manuscript; and all authors approved the final manuscript as submitted.

doi:10.1542/peds.2013-2521

Opting in to Online Professionalism: Social Media and Pediatrics

INTRODUCTORY COMMENTARY

The Council on Medical Student Education in Pediatrics (COMSEP) is committed to excellence in medical student education in pediatrics. This article continues our series on skills of, and strategies used by, great clinical teachers. Kind et al argue that the digital world provides a great opportunity for clinical educators to promote and enhance student education and model professionalism. They provide resources and tips to get started using this domain.

—Susan Bannister, MD

Editor-in-Chief, COMSEP Monthly Feature

Social media can be described as a digital space for creating and sharing information with others, disseminating it widely and rapidly.[1] It can extend real-life learning and relationships into a shared space to foster online connections and learning. Physicians and physicians-in-training are entering this digital environment with little guidance on best practices. Professionalism

lapses online can have consequences not only for individuals but also for public trust in the medical profession.[2] And yet, when used well, social media enriches the personal and professional lives of clinicians and learners. We'll consider the risky (red) zone, the safe but go slow (yellow) zone, and the opt in to opportunity (green) zone to explain the challenges students may face and to outline how to teach and model professionalism in the use of social media.

WHERE AND HOW ARE PEOPLE CONNECTING ON SOCIAL MEDIA?

Several studies describe social media use by medical students,[3,4] physicians,[5,6] and medical educators.[7] In 2012, 67% of online adults reported using Facebook, 20% LinkedIn, 16% Twitter, 15% Pinterest, 13% Instagram, and 6% Tumblr.[8,9] These and other platforms allow users to connect through words, photos, audio, or videos in various ways: privately or publicly, synchronously or asynchronously, and uni- or multidirectionally.

There are also less public avenues, such as secure or physician-only networks where credentials are verified, such as Doximity, QuantiaMD, Sermo, and forMD. The decision to use an invitation-only, secure forum or a more publicly available domain depends on one's goals.

THE GUIDELINES: MAINTAINING ONLINE PROFESSIONALISM

Organizations, including the American Medical Association (AMA),[2] the Canadian Medical Association,[10] the Federation of State Medical Boards,[11] and some medical schools,[12] have guidelines regarding professionalism in the use of social media, emphasizing pitfalls and benefits of engagement.[13] Modeling and teaching this dimension of professionalism, online, digital, or e-professionalism, is increasingly important.[14] The AMA recommends that physicians with a social media presence maintain patient privacy, routinely monitor their presence, maintain appropriate boundaries just as they would in other contexts, consider separating personal from professional, and recognize the impact their actions and those of their colleagues can have on public trust.[2]

Although social media use with patients is beyond the scope of this brief piece, we note that the American Academy of Pediatrics has recognized the impact of social media on pediatric patients and families,[15] and an extensive review of the ethical implications of social media and clinical care was recently published.[16] Many pediatric patients and medical students have grown up with technology and are comfortable in the social medial realm. Clinical educators benefit from understanding the online challenges and opportunities presented by social media and, by modeling professional behaviors, they can assist their students in exchanging ideas and learning to use social media safely and professionally.

ONLINE AND OFFLINE

Just as one's online identity can be appraised in the context of one's offline identity, online professionalism may be seen in the context of traditional tenets of professionalism in pediatrics. Clinical teachers must recognize what platform they are on, how public it is, and who is welcome; they also need to know when to listen, when to contribute, what relationships to forge, and when to point out how others might behave more professionally.

RED ZONE: RISKS

Breaching patient privacy on social media (and offline) is unacceptable. Because digital content is highly accessible, easily disseminated, and often indelible, professionalism lapses online can loom large. Users must be aware of and heed their employer's, hospital's, or school's policies. Opting

for anonymity is risky because one may not truly be anonymous. Moreover, physicians posting with or without their names still risk diminishing public trust in the profession, particularly if they are perceived as unprofessional (eg, if depicted as intoxicated, using profanity, and/or making disparaging remarks about patients).

YELLOW ZONE: CAN BE SAFE IF YOU GO SLOW

Clinical educators should develop their own rationale for online interactions with learners, colleagues, and/or patients and be aware of the public nature of these interactions. Tips include the following: having separate accounts or using different platforms for the personal and the professional, thinking before you post, using humor cautiously, and recognizing and managing your digital footprint.

GREEN ZONE: BENEFITS AND OPPORTUNITIES TO ADD VALUE

Positive uses include disseminating accurate information, countering posted inaccuracies, modeling professionalism (including explicitly protecting patient privacy), and engaging learners and the public outside traditional classrooms or offices (Table 1). Share research, network, and find out what else is going on in pediatrics. Tweeting at a meeting is a way to reflect-in-action, share questions publicly, and find others with similar interests. Online, you can mentor and be mentored.[17] Consider joining an online community (chat) or using social media to augment traditional teaching such as with flipped classroom techniques.[18]

PROMOTING PROFESSIONALISM AMONG STUDENTS

By being responsible and professional in one's own social media use, or by recognizing challenges and opportunities,

TABLE 1 Questions to Guide Your Social Media "Action Plan" as a Pediatric Educator

Reflect on your own social media identity
- Who were you, who are you now, and how would you like to portray yourself?
- Who do you represent when online?
- What content will you share? What value will you add?
- How will you separate the personal from the professional?

Your social media goals, actions, and opportunities
- What do you aim to do on social media? What do you want to learn more about?
- Will you contribute educational content? Will you participate in a chat? Are there topics you wish to address in an online community?
- How can you enhance your use of social media for public good?
- What is your plan for next steps? Will you observe/listen, join, participate, contribute?
- How will you use technology to help you communicate, collaborate, and connect? Will you mentor others? Teach and learn? Engage in and promote reflection?

Your social media interactions
- With whom will you connect? Students (past or present), residents, colleagues, and/or patients? Who/what are the people, topics, and/or organizations you affiliate with?
- When will you interact in a secure, private online space, and when in a open forum?
- How will you interact? One to one, one to many, or multidirectionally? Synchronously or asynchronously? Will this complement face-to-face interaction?

Caveats
- How will you ensure patient privacy?
- How will you maintain professionalism?
- How will you navigate relationships (new and preexisting)? What tone will you use? How will you provide feedback about professionalism to others?

Promoting professionalism among your students
- How will you promote online professionalism, and who will mentor the students?
- What will you do when you see unprofessional social media content by your students?
- How can you show that the principles of professionalism offline apply online as well?

clinical teachers can serve as mentors for students. Invite discourse when opportunities arise (eg, when you see questionable posts by physicians or physicians-in-training or controversial news reports involving social media), and engage in discussions with students using real or hypothetical cases, rather than blocking their social media access altogether. If you come across unprofessional content by your students, you should bring it to their attention, ask for their analysis of the professional implications, encourage reflection, and help them recognize potential consequences of their actions. Residents may be involved as near-peer mentors for students regarding responsible social media use because they may be closer in age and attitude.[17]

GOALS DRIVE SOCIAL MEDIA USE

If as a clinical educator your goal is to develop a resource guide for students, a wiki where multiple contributors can update entries would work well. If you want to foster reflective practice among students, secure invitation-only blogs, where learners post and comment on one another's reflections are good choices. If you want to counter inaccuracies, you could have students find misinformation about a topic (eg, vaccination) and create a "myth-busting" blog post or YouTube video. If your goal is to chat openly across medical specialties throughout the country (and world), a live/synchronous chat on Twitter may be the answer. Or, individual physicians may look to secure "verified" physician-only networks as the best option to discuss pediatric care–related questions with other physicians.

SELECTED RESOURCES

- Pew Internet and American Life Project (www.pewinternet.org):

descriptive statistics on how people use social media, including for health.

- Medical education (www.twitter. com/MedEdChat) and other health care–related tweet chats (www. symplur.com/healthcare-hashtags/ tweet-chats): Tweet chats are open, synchronous, virtual conversations on Twitter, prearranged to occur at recurring time periods. Predefined hashtags index the content (eg, #meded for medical education–related discussions).

- Social media outlets from the American Association of Medical Colleges (https://www.aamc.org/about/follow): explore how the American Association of Medical Colleges uses social media for discussion among applicants, students, residents, physician-educators, and advisors.

- The AMA on professionalism in the use of social media (http://www. ama-assn.org/ama/pub/physician-resources/medical-ethics/code-medical-ethics/opinion9124.page): physicians should be aware of these ethical considerations when maintaining an online presence.

CONCLUSIONS

Increasingly, students will have grown up interacting through social media well before they become professional adults. It is the clinical educator's responsibility to help them apply principles of professionalism that exist offline to the online arena. One way to better understand and help is to opt in to responsible social media use, being cognizant of pitfalls as well as opportunities to connect, learn, teach, and model professionalism. Another way is to engage in explicit discussion with students, sharing examples of responsible social media use and critiquing examples of irresponsible social media use. If you feel stuck at

the red light, skeptical about commingling social media and your career, first explore and observe. Soon you will want to move with the traffic, get into the green zone and opt in online, modeling professionalism and making productive use of social media.

ACKNOWLEDGMENTS

The authors thank Dr Katherine Chretien for her thoughtful discussions and Drs Robert Dudas, Janice Hanson, and Susan Bannister for their suggestions and editing.

REFERENCES

1. Greysen SR, Kind T, Chretien KC. Online professionalism and the mirror of social media. *J Gen Intern Med.* 2010;25(11):1227–1229

2. Shore R, Halsey J, Shah K, Crigger BJ, Douglas SP; AMA Council on Ethical and Judicial Affairs (CEJA). Report of the AMA Council on Ethical and Judicial Affairs: professionalism in the use of social media. *J Clin Ethics.* 2011;22(2):165–172

3. Chretien KC, Greysen SR, Chretien JP, Kind T. Online posting of unprofessional content by medical students. *JAMA.* 2009;302(12): 1309–1315

4. Lie DA, Trial JT, Schaff P, Wallace R, Elliott D. "Being the best we can be": medical students' reflections on physician responsibility in the social media era. *Acad Med.* 2013;88(2):240–245

5. Chretien KC, Azar J, Kind T. Physicians on Twitter. *JAMA.* 2011;305(6):566–568

6. McGowan BS, Wasko M, Vartabedian BS, Miller RS, Freiherr DD, Abdolrasulnia M. Understanding the factors that influence the adoption and meaningful use of social media by physicians to share medical information. *J Med Internet Res.* 2012;14(5): e117

7. Kind T, Greysen SR, Chretien KC. Pediatric clerkship directors' social networking use and perceptions of online professionalism. *Acad Pediatr.* 2012;12(2):142–148

8. Madden M, Zickuhr K. 65% of online adults use social networking sites. Pew Internet & American Life Project, Aug 26, 2011. Available at: http://pewinternet.org/Reports/2011/Social-Networking-Sites.aspx. Accessed April 1, 2013

9. Brenner J. Pew Internet: social networking (full detail). Pew Internet & American Life Project, Feb 14, 2013. Available at: http://

pewinternet.org/Commentary/2012/March/ Pew-Internet-Social-Networking-full-detail.aspx. Accessed April 1, 2013

10. Federation of State Medical Boards. Model policy guidelines for the appropriate use of social media and social networking in medical practice. Available at: www.fsmb.org/pdf/ pub-social-media-guidelines.pdf. Accessed July 10, 2013

11. Canadian Medical Association. Social media and Canadian physicians—issues and rules of engagement. Available at: www.cma. ca/advocacy/social-media-canadian-physicians. Accessed July 10, 2013

12. Kind T, Genrich G, Sodhi A, Chretien KC. Social media policies at US medical schools. *Med Educ Online.* 2010;15. doi: 10.3402/meo.v15i0.5324.

13. Kind T, Greysen SR, Chretien KC. Advantages and challenges of social media in pediatrics. *Pediatr Ann.* 2011;40(9):430–434

14. Kaczmarczyk JM, Chuang A, Dugoff L, et al. e-Professionalism: a new frontier in medical education. *Teach Learn Med.* 2013;25(2): 165–170

15. O'Keeffe GS, Clarke-Pearson K; Council on Communications and Media. The impact of social media on children, adolescents, and families. *Pediatrics.* 2011;127(4):800–804

16. Chretien KC, Kind T. Social media and clinical care: ethical, professional, and social implications. *Circulation.* 2013;127(13):1413–1421

17. Patel PD, Roberts JL, Miller KH, Ziegler C, Ostapchuk M. The responsible use of online social networking: who should mentor medical students. *Teach Learn Med.* 2012; 24(4):348–354

18. Khan S. Let's use video to reinvent education. TED: Ideas Worth Spreading. 2011. Available at: www.ted.com/talks/salman_ khan_let_s_use_video_to_reinvent_education. html. Accessed April 1, 2013

FINANCIAL DISCLOSURE: The authors have indicated they have no financial relationships relevant to this article to disclose.
FUNDING: No external funding.
POTENTIAL CONFLICT OF INTEREST: The authors have indicated they have no potential conflicts of interest to disclose.

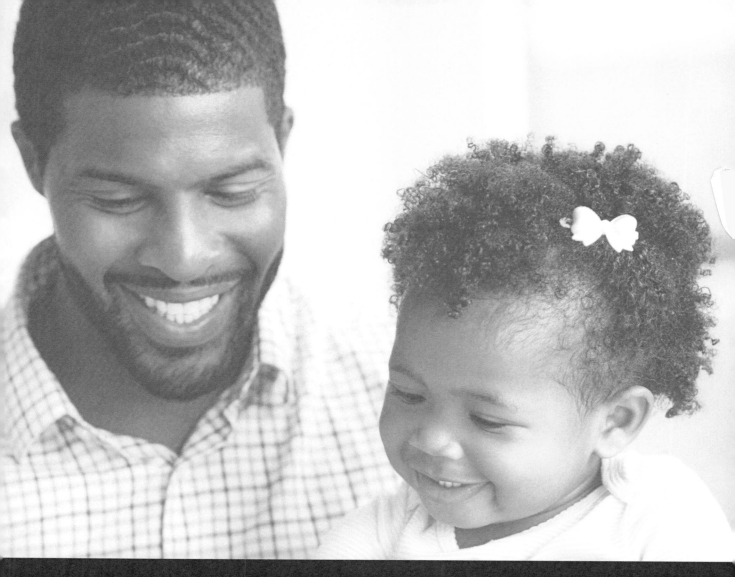

Chapter 7: Trust & Decision Making

Chapter 7

The Value of Trusting Relationships in Shared Decision Making

By Christopher G Maloney, MD, PhD
Professor, Department of Pediatrics, University of Nebraska College of Medicine

The great clinical teacher strives to impart knowledge and skills to learners and model effective patient and family-centered communication. Of critical importance is building trusting relationships, and it is with trust that shared decision making is enabled and fostered.

A hallmark of pediatric primary care is well child care. Parents look to their pediatrician to provide advice on growth, development, nutrition, and other issues.[1] However, there may be other more important sensitive issues that parents seek advice on that may not come to light without first establishing trust and the space to share concerns. For example, without trust, will the mother of your patient share her feelings of postpartum depression or being in a physically abusive relationship? Will disparities in terms of social determinants of health be disclosed?[2,3] Will concerns about transportation, financial stress, and taking time off work for clinical appointments[3] come up in discussion? There is no doubt that by knowing about the issues their patients are facing, clinicians are better able to develop a management plan that will work for the patient and family. But how does the clinical educator teach this to their learners?

In the first of this chapter's COMSEP articles, Balog et al describe tools to support effective communication during well child visits. The first strategy described is "Elicit and ask...then assess, prioritize, and advise," an approach that aims to focus on the family's concerns and meet their needs, recognizing that concerns may need to be elicited several times during a visit to uncover more sensitive issues as rapport is developed. Similarly, the CHEC(k)-UP tool (Concerns, History, Environment, Child, Unanswered questions, and Prioritized anticipatory guidance) prioritizes patient concerns first and at the end of the visit. These tools, along with reliable resources such as the AAP's Bright Futures website (brightfutures.aap.org) to guide anticipatory guidance[4] can help provide learners with communication strategies and a framework to develop trusting relationships and align their agenda with that of the patient and family and thus contribute to shared decision making.

Shared decision making is essential in clinical educational contexts beyond well child care visits. There is much attention on the importance of high-value care, eliminating practices and associated expenditures that are not evidence-based and do not directly benefit patients; this too can be role-modeled by the clinical teacher. High-value care is defined by the 2013 Institute of Medicine report as "the best care for the patient, with the optimal result for the circumstances, delivered at the right price."[5] Building trusting relationships influences communication to effectively share decision making to improve value.

Tools in the teacher's toolbox are described in the article by Volpe Holmes et al and include PPI (Prepare, Process and Initiate) and SOAP-V, adding "Value" to the traditional Subjective, Objective, Assessment and Plan narrative.[6] PPI teaches the learner to understand overdiagnosis[7] and the unintentional effects a laboratory result may have on additional work-up or treatment. SOAP-V relies on the definition of value, asking what is the improvement in quality, safety, or experience relative to cost of the intervention.[8] Furthermore, both tools enhance shared decision making with families when trusting relationships exist.

Shared decision making can come to fruition only when a trusting relationship is established between the patient and family and the clinician. Whether in the context of well child care or making clinical decisions that are guided by principles of high-value care, the clinical teacher can role model and provide guidance to learners so they, too, can develop trusting relationships with their patients and families.

References

1. Schor EL. Rethinking well-child care. Pediatrics. Jul 2004;114(1):210-6. doi:10.1542/peds.114.1.210.
2. Thornton RL, Glover CM, Cené CW, Glik DC, Henderson JA, Williams DR. Evaluating Strategies For Reducing Health Disparities By Addressing The Social Determinants Of Health. *Health Aff (Millwood)*. 08 2016;35(8):1416-23. doi:10.1377/hlthaff.2015.1357.
3. Wolf ER, O'Neil J, Pecsok J, et al. Caregiver and Clinician Perspectives on Missed Well-Child Visits. *Ann Fam Med*. 01 2020;18(1):30-34. doi:10.1370/afm.2466.
4. Balog EK, Hanson JL, Blaschke GS. Teaching the essentials of "well-child care": inspiring proficiency and passion. *Pediatrics*. Aug 2014;134(2):206-9. doi:10.1542/peds.2014-1372.
5. Creating a New Culture of Care. In: Medicine Io, ed. Best Care at Lower Cost: The Path to Continuously Learning Health Care in America. The National Academies Press; 2013:255-280.
6. Volpe Holmes A, Long M, Stallworth J. We Can Teach How to Bend the Cost Curve: Lessons in Pediatric High-Value Health Care. *Pediatrics*. 03 2017;139(3)doi:10.1542/peds.2016-4016.
7. Coon ER, Quinonez RA, Moyer VA, Schroeder AR. Overdiagnosis: how our compulsion for diagnosis may be harming children. *Pediatrics*. Nov 2014;134(5):1013-23. doi:10.1542/peds.2014-1778.
8. Smith A, Andrews S, Wilkins V, De Beritto T, Jenkins S, Maloney CG. Value Narratives: A Novel Method for Understanding High-Cost Pediatric Hospital Patients. *Hosp Pediatr*. 10 2016;6(10):569-577. doi:10.1542/hpeds.2016-0033.

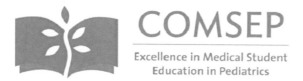

AUTHORS: Erin K. Balog, MD,[a] Janice L. Hanson, PhD,[b] and Gregory S. Blaschke, MD, MPH[c]

[a]Department of Pediatrics, Uniformed Services University of the Health Sciences, Bethesda, Maryland; [b]Department of Pediatrics, University of Colorado School of Medicine, Aurora, Colorado; and [c]Department of Pediatrics, Oregon Health and Sciences University, Portland, Oregon

Address correspondence to Erin K. Balog, MD, CDR, MC, USN, Department of Pediatrics, Uniformed Services University of the Health Sciences. E-mail: erin.balog@usuhs.edu

Accepted for publication May 9, 2014

KEY WORDS
clinical teacher, medical student

Dr Balog wrote the original first draft of the article, did most of the re-drafting of the article, and sought, read, and reviewed all the references; Drs Hanson and Blaschke contributed much of the content to the outline of the first draft of the article, and assisted with multiple re-drafts of the article; and all authors approved the final manuscript as submitted.

The views expressed in this article are those of the author and do not reflect the official policy or position of the US Navy, Department of Defense, or the US Government.

doi:10.1542/peds.2014-1372

Teaching the Essentials of "Well-Child Care": Inspiring Proficiency and Passion

Before the pediatric clerkship, most medical students learn to take a patient history starting with the "chief complaint." Upon encountering their first pediatric patients, students quickly recognize that they are not prepared to ask the appropriate follow-up questions when the chief complaint is "well-child visit." In this article, we present a practical method for teaching medical students how to approach pediatric health supervision visits that build upon their existing clinical skills.

Primary care pediatricians address the health care needs of each child in the context of their family and community. They acknowledge the important ways in which social and psychological determinants of health impact wellness. Clinical teachers of pediatrics can inspire future physicians to use patient-centered communication skills to address the needs and priorities of families by making explicit the different aspects of a pediatric health supervision visit that include the following:

1. Identifying patient and family concerns by practicing a structured communication strategy.

2. Using reliable resources to identify the established priorities for each age and access most up-to-date anticipatory guidance recommendations.

3. Delivering prioritized anticipatory guidance that is specific to each patient within his or her community.

COMMUNICATION STRATEGY

A useful strategy for approaching the conversation with parents and children is for students to: "Elicit and ask...then assess, prioritize, and advise."[1] Clinical preceptors should explain the importance of eliciting patient and family concerns by asking open-ended questions. Then, with feedback on their ability to assess the most important issues, preceptors ask students to prioritize which topics to

address and then together, advise the family accordingly.

Eliciting concerns through open-ended questions creates the essential foundation for the health supervision visit.[2] Recent studies have demonstrated that using a patient-centered communication style with open-ended questions is not only time-effective but allows for greater adherence to the current standards for well-child care practice.[2,3] If "closed-ended" or "leading questions" are used, the student risks neglecting the family's concerns and may deliver advice that does not meet the needs of their patients.[4] In fact, students often need to elicit concerns several times during the encounter because the more sensitive concerns such as financial insecurity or family discord are frequently uncovered after the student builds rapport.[5] We direct students to use the acronym CHEC (k)-UP[1] when taking a complete history for a well-child visit that prioritizes obtaining the patient concerns first and again at the end of the visit:

C   -Concerns (or questions)
H   -History (past medical, birth, family, social)
E   -Environment (home, typical day, nutrition, sleep)
C   -Child (development, growth, voiding)
U   -Unanswered questions (inquire about further concerns)
P   -Prioritized anticipatory guidance

Although the components of a "complete history" are familiar to students, the specific components of a health supervision history may be new to them. In particular, pediatricians can explain the tenets of collecting a developmental history that includes surveillance as well as formal screening.[6] Table 1 contains a list of possible open-ended questions that we developed for students to use. The first question listed in the table can be used to open the visit so that family and patient concerns are collected up front. Students can also be taught to ask questions that highlight family and patient strengths in addition to uncovering risk factors. For example, "What new things is your child doing?" instead of "Is your child using at least fifty words?"[7]

After completing the history and a physical examination, students should organize their data and synthesize an assessment of the visit by presenting a concise oral presentation.[8] After discussing these interpretations with their preceptor, students should make an attempt to prioritize the topics for anticipatory guidance and either observe their preceptor or directly advise or counsel the patient and family themselves.

RELIABLE RESOURCES

In 2008, the American Academy of Pediatrics published a new set of health supervision guidelines, *Bright Futures: Guidelines for Health Supervision of Infants, Children, and Adolescents, third edition.* [2] This edition includes the text, a pocket guide along with a tool, and

resource kit for implementation. Students can access the pocket guide version of this text electronically.[9] The overarching themes are listed below:

	Bright Futures Themes Promoting...
• Family support	• Physical activity
• Child development	• Oral health
• Mental health	• Healthy sexual development and sexuality
• Healthy weight	• Safety and injury prevention
• Healthy nutrition	• Community relationships and resources

The Bright Futures Pocket Guide provides a "menu" of 5 possible anticipatory guidance topics for each age from newborn to age 21, such as an introduction to oral health at 6 months of age

and developmental and mental health assessment for children 8 years of age.[9] Students can self-identify knowledge gaps related to these common anticipatory guidance topics. For example, a student may choose to learn more about effective discipline, early literacy, or car seat safety by accessing trustworthy parental resources online such as www.caringforkids.cps.ca, www.cdc.gov/parents, or www.healthychildren.org.

ANTICIPATORY GUIDANCE

Before the first encounter, clinical teachers should clearly convey their expectations so that students know whether to address concerns independently or wait until they have reviewed their approach with the preceptor. Pediatricians should explain to students how they identify

TABLE 1 Open-ended Questions for Well-Child Visits: Key Topics and *Bright Futures* Themes

Key Topics for Anticipatory Guidance	Bright Futures Themes[2]
Patient and family concerns	
What concerns or questions would you like to cover today?	Family-centered communication
Home	
Who lives at home?	Family support
Who among your friends and family provides support to you?	
What recent changes have happened at home?	
Day/night/routines	
Where does your child spend the day?	
What opportunities does your child have for active play and exercise?	Physical activity
How has your child adjusted to daycare/preschool/school?	Mental health
What questions or concerns do you have about your child's progress or performance in school?	Child development
What is your child's bedtime routine?	Safety and injury prevention
What questions or concerns do you have about your child's sleep?	
Diet/nutrition	
What kinds of foods does your child eat?	Healthy nutrition
How do you feed your child?	Healthy weight
What questions or concerns do you have about your child's eating?	
Development/behavior	
What new things is your child doing?	Child development
What questions or concerns do you have about your child's growth or development?	Mental health
What questions or concerns do you have about your child's behavior?	Healthy sexual development and sexuality
How do you encourage your child?	
How do you discipline your child?	
Oral health	
How do you care for your child's teeth?	Oral health
Safety	
How have you made your home safe for your children?	Safety and injury prevention
How do you ensure your child's safety in the car?	

the most important advice for each individual patient and family based on their personal knowledge of the child and understanding of the community context in which that child lives. For example, clinical teachers can explain how they choose to target injury prevention based on the rural, suburban, or urban context of the patients in their communities: Pool safety might be prioritized for a child learning to swim in the summer, whereas the occupational hazards related to heavy machinery and animals would be reserved for children who live on a farm.

Students should avoid using the *Bright Futures Pocket Guide* as a "checklist" of items to complete because patients and families are likely to only recall a fraction of what is discussed.[10] In fact, *Bright Futures* is not meant to be a checklist but a guide or menu of options that allow the provider to select items within each domain to match the needs of the patient, provider, and communities (G. Blaschke, MD, MPH, personal communication, 2014). Providers demonstrate the principles of prioritization by identifying and addressing individual patient concerns while balancing what is known about health promotion, injury prevention, and the strengths and needs of the community. In addition, when providers acknowledge and support the family who knows that child best, long-term relationship building can be modeled effectively.

Most students at this stage in their training are likely to require guidance on how to effectively influence behavior change using patient-centered interview techniques.[11] Behavior change, such as tobacco cessation or alcohol and drug screening in adolescents, can be facilitated with motivational interviewing and brief interventions.[4] Preceptors can help teach the basics of these skills by asking students to practice sharing information about one

of the prioritized topics by role-playing a parent or older child while the student attempts to offer them advice.[12] Advanced students may also be able to identify barriers to implementation and assess whether the family has accurately understood the information.[13] Student communication skills can further improve when a clinical teacher "debriefs" with the student after the visit by explicitly describing the process that guided his or her actions during the consultation.[14]

When students are able to access reliable resources for information, they are better equipped to self-identify knowledge gaps and practice delivering prioritized advice with supervision. By using the "Elicit and ask...then assess, prioritize, and advise" patient-centered communication strategy, students learn to balance "their" agenda with the agenda of the patient and family. With a few weeks of supervised practice, students learn to address each patient's most pressing needs and provide advice that is informed by evidence and specifically targeted to each patient in the context of their family and community. Moreover, students are likely to overcome their initial "fears" of pediatric patients whereby they can come to enjoy the moments that bring families back to their trusted partner who supports the care for their developing child.

ACKNOWLEDGMENTS

Dr Balog led the process of rewrites with the Council on Medical Student Education in Pediatrics editorial committee, which included Dr Susan Bannister and Dr Robert Dudas. COMSEP supported this project with an educational scholarship grant in 2009.

REFERENCES

1. Hanson J, Balog E, Pelzner M. Pediatric health supervision curriculum: Instructor's guide, student resources, faculty resources, and assessment tools. *MedEdPORTAL.*
2014. Available at: www.mededportal.org/publication/9752. Accessed June 1, 2014

2. Hagan JFSJ, Duncan PM, eds. *Bright Futures: Guidelines for Health Supervision of Infants, Children, and Adolescents,* 3rd ed. Elk Grove Village, IL: American Academy of Pediatrics; 2008

3. Norlin C, Crawford MA, Bell CT, Sheng X, Stein MT. Delivery of well-child care: a look inside the door. *Acad Pediatr.* 2011;11(1):18–26

4. Barnes AJ, Gold MA. Promoting healthy behaviors in pediatrics: motivational interviewing. *Pediatrics in Review.* 2012;33(9). Available at: www.pediatrics.org/cgi/content/full/33/9/e57

5. Epstein RM, Mauksch L, Carroll J, Jaén CR. Have you really addressed your patient's concerns? *Fam Pract Manag.* 2008;15(3):35–40

6. Council on Children With Disabilities; Section on Developmental Behavioral Pediatrics; Bright Futures Steering Committee; Medical Home Initiatives for Children With Special Needs Project Advisory Committee. Identifying infants and young children with developmental disorders in the medical home: an algorithm for developmental surveillance and screening. *Pediatrics.* 2006;118(1):405–420

7. Committee on Hospital Care and Institute for Patient- and Family-Centered Care. Patient- and family-centered care and the pediatrician's role. *Pediatrics.* 2012;129(2):394–404

8. Dell M, Lewin L, Gigante J. What's the story? Expectations for oral case presentations. *Pediatrics.* 2012;130(1):1–4

9. *Bright Futures Pocket Guide.* Elk Grove Village, IL: American Academy of Pediatrics; 2008. Available at: https://brightfutures.aap.org/pdfs/BF3%20pocket%20guide_final.pdf. Accessed June 1, 2014

10. Barkin SL, Scheindlin B, Brown C, Ip E, Finch S, Wasserman RC. Anticipatory guidance topics: are more better? *Ambul Pediatr.* 2005;5(6):372–376

11. White LL, Gazewood JD, Mounsey AL. Teaching students behavior change skills: description and assessment of a new Motivational interviewing curriculum. *Med Teach.* 2007;29(4):e67–e71

12. Mounsey AL, Bovbjerg V, White L, Gazewood J. Do students develop better motivational interviewing skills through role-play with standardised patients or with student colleagues? *Med Educ.* 2006;40(8):775–780

13. Bell K, Cole BA. Improving medical students' success in promoting health behavior change:

a curriculum evaluation. *J Gen Intern Med.* 2008;23(9):1503–1506

14. Cruess SR, Cruess RL, Steinert Y. Role modelling—making the most of a powerful teaching strategy. *BMJ.* 2008;336(7646):718–721

FINANCIAL DISCLOSURE: The authors have indicated they have no financial relationships relevant to this article to disclose.
FUNDING: Funding for this project was supported by a COMSEP Educational Research Grant in 2009.
POTENTIAL CONFLICT OF INTEREST: The authors have indicated they have no potential conflicts of interest to disclose.

We Can Teach How to Bend the Cost Curve: Lessons in Pediatric High-Value Health Care

Alison Volpe Holmes, MD, MPH,[a,b,c] Michele Long, MD,[d,e] James Stallworth, MD[f]

"We have really good data that show when you take patients and you really inform them about their choices, patients make more frugal choices. They pick more efficient choices than the health care system does."

Donald Berwick, MD

In continuing the series of articles by the Council on Medical Student Education in Pediatrics, we focus on the great clinical teacher's responsibility to both deliver and explicitly teach about high-value health care. Medical students entering clinical rotations have been introduced to the concept of "too much care" in their coursework, including overdiagnosis, overtreatment, excessive testing, and poor care coordination and communication.[1,2] As pediatricians committed to eliminating practices and associated expenditures that are not evidence-based and that lack direct patient benefit, we can improve our clinical teaching skills by making our role-modeling of such behaviors explicit. This paper reviews ways to incorporate teaching about common examples of pediatric care of limited or no value by using accessible teaching tools, such as the Choosing Wisely lists.[3] We also introduce 2 efficient teaching aids to help learners incorporate the concept of value into their clinical reasoning and presentations: Prepare, Process, Initiate (PPI), and Subjective,

Objective, Assessment, Plan, Value (SOAP-V).[4]

EXCESSIVE COSTS OF HEALTH CARE IN THE UNITED STATES: PROPORTION FROM "TOO MUCH CARE"

Despite the modest deceleration in the rate of rise in total US health care expenditures over the last few years, health care spending in the United States vastly exceeds spending in other developed nations, yet our health outcomes are worse.[5] The societal impact is substantial: health care indebtedness is the leading cause of household bankruptcy, and increasing health insurance premiums have eliminated real growth in wages for the past 2 decades.[6,7] "Too much" care also comes at a personal cost to patients and families, including side effects from unneeded medications and complications from unnecessary procedures.

Approximately half of excess health care cost due to various categories of "waste" in the health care system falls into domains that are under the control of physicians.[2] These include failures of care delivery and coordination, and wasteful excessive care in the form of overdiagnosis, overtesting, and overtreatment. Although pediatrics is not typically viewed as a source of excessive

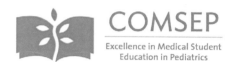

[a]Department of Pediatrics, Geisel School of Medicine at Dartmouth, Hanover, New Hampshire; [b]Children's Hospital at Dartmouth-Hitchcock, Lebanon, New Hampshire; [c]The Dartmouth Institute, Lebanon, New Hampshire; [d]Department of Pediatrics, School of Medicine, and [e]UCSF Benioff Children's Hospital, University of California San Francisco, San Francisco, California; and [f]Division of General Pediatrics, Department of Pediatrics, University of South Carolina School of Medicine, Columbia, South Carolina

Dr Holmes conceptualized and designed the article, wrote the initial version, and reviewed and revised the manuscript; Dr Long helped with conceptualization of the manuscript, was the primary author of the table, and reviewed and revised the manuscript; Dr Stallworth helped with conceptualization of the manuscript, developed the Prepare, Process, Initiate model, and reviewed and revised the manuscript; and all authors approved the final manuscript as submitted.

DOI: 10.1542/peds.2016-4016

Accepted for publication Nov 30, 2016

Address correspondence to Alison Volpe Holmes, MD, MPH, 1 Medical Center Dr, Rubin 525, Lebanon, NH 03756. E-mail: alison.v.holmes@hitchcock.org

PEDIATRICS (ISSN Numbers: Print, 0031-4005; Online, 1098-4275).

FINANCIAL DISCLOSURE: The authors have indicated they have no financial relationships relevant to this article to disclose.

FUNDING: No external funding.

POTENTIAL CONFLICT OF INTEREST: The authors have indicated they have no potential conflicts of interest to disclose.

To cite: Holmes AV, Long M, Stallworth J. We Can Teach How to Bend the Cost Curve: Lessons in Pediatric High-Value Health Care. *Pediatrics.* 2017;139(3):e20164016

costs, significant opportunities for value improvement in pediatrics exist, and pediatric costs are rising faster than costs in adult health service delivery.[8,9] Many students who complete pediatric rotations eventually pursue other specialties, but the principles of high-value care are readily transferable.

WHY TEACH ABOUT HEALTH CARE VALUE?

Given the excessive costs in US health care and their effects on patients and families, value and quality require more explicit emphasis in our pediatric teaching. Traditional clinical reasoning instruction results in the generation of extensive and frequently exhaustive differential diagnoses for common presenting complaints. This can have the unintended effect of teaching students and residents that no diagnostic possibility should go unexplored.[10] Although limiting premature diagnostic closure and ensuring consideration of an accurate differential diagnosis are critical, sound clinical reasoning is also compatible with the teaching of restraint, stepwise decision-making, plans that avoid excess, and the incorporation of patient and family perspectives. When exploring clinical reasoning of learners, we can ask them to explain both the utility and the risks of tests they would like to order.[5,10] Clinical teachers should explain the complexity, work, and unintended consequences of potential false positive results , even for what seem like "simple" tests. Although students who accurately identify a rare diagnosis receive praise, we rarely reward those who arrive at appropriate assessments with limited testing and consultation, or those who are comfortable with the uncertainty of waiting for the first round of limited testing to return, or observing a patient for a few days to see if improvement occurs. Noting and praising these behaviors more frequently could, over time, move our training culture toward high-value care.[4,10]

TOOLS FOR TEACHING HIGH-VALUE CARE

Choosing Wisely is a public education campaign whose purpose is to begin conversations between patients and physicians about potentially unnecessary tests and treatments. It highlights specific targets for improving value in pediatric primary care, inpatient, nursery, and select subspecialty settings, providing an excellent starting point for teaching basic pediatric high-value care. Pediatricians should have familiarity with these recommendations and potentially post them in their workrooms, or on course Web sites for easy access by learners and for use in teaching. These resources, which include references and evidence supporting all recommendations, are available at: www.choosingwisely.org.

Clinical teachers should role model honest conversations with families about current evidence-based decision-making, calculated risks versus benefits, and areas of uncertainty in clinical knowledge and practice. By doing so, they engage patients and parents in shared decision-making, and patients will often choose the less invasive, less aggressive approach.[11]

PPI AND SOAP-V MODELS FOR CLINICAL ENCOUNTERS

PPI is a newly proposed and practical approach for teaching learners to apply the concepts of high-value care in pediatrics. Before a patient encounter, oral presentation, or before writing a note, the preceptor communicates with the learner using the following tool:

"Prepare": What are the benefits versus harms of testing, interventions, and treatments related to the presenting problem, in general, but also, more specifically, to this particular patient?

"Process": What evidence exists pertaining to the presenting problem and the proposed interventions?

"Initiate": Of the interventions available, which ones will maximize benefit, minimize harm, and be least costly? Here, preceptors emphasize to learners that patients and parents should share in this decision-making.

See Table 1 for examples of how the PPI model applies to common pediatric conditions.

SOAP-V adds "value" to the traditional Subjective-Objective-Assessment-Plan presentation by incorporating 3 value elements in the framing of management plans.[4] Ask students to include answers to these questions when presenting a plan: (1) Does adding my proposed intervention potentially change management? Does it meaningfully benefit the patient? (2) Have I incorporated patient and family values and circumstances, and considered potential harms? (3) What is known about the cost of the intervention, both immediately and downstream?

VALUE AND ETHICS

Lessons on the principle of nonmaleficence (primum non nocere) are abundantly available in the teaching of high-value care. Although the bioethical principle of beneficence has led some to believe that cost should never be a consideration in treatment decisions, Schroeder and Ralston[18] have recently illustrated how the bioethical principle of parsimony entreats us to effectively diagnose and treat each patient in the most efficient manner possible, with the efficient approach containing the most benefit for the patient.

TABLE 1 Using PPI To Teach Value

Setting	Example	Prepare	Process	Initiate
Office	Parents of a thriving 4-mo-old infant ask if she needs medications for her "reflux."	Could acid suppressing medication help? Are there harms?	Systematic review of articles on acid suppression harms and Choosing Wisely show no benefit and increased risk of infections.[3,12]	Reassure family that spit-up is normal if growth is fine; come to shared decision not to use medication.
Office	An immunized 18-mo-old child has a normal neurologic exam and a viral exanthem after a simple febrile seizure.	Does this child need more work-up for seizures? Is there potential harm from a CT scan?	AAN/AAP guideline and Choosing Wisely: no EEG or head imaging needed. Consider potential harms of radiation, sedation, inadvertent findings.[3,13]	Empathize with family on how frightening this was, but explain how it is also common and the absence of long-term effects. Counsel what to do if there is a recurrence.
Office	A low-risk, 120-h-old, 41-wk gestation girl has a serum bilirubin of 20.1 mg/dL. Mother reports her milk is in, and baby has gained 20 g since the previous day.	Should we initiate phototherapy? Are there side effects to phototherapy, such as impact on bonding?	Measured level is below the AAP guideline phototherapy line; NNT in this category is >3000.[14,15]	Discuss risks/harms of phototherapy and treatment alternatives, such as a repeat bilirubin level the next day and continued frequent breastfeeding in a comfortable home setting.
ED	A 3-y-old girl presents with minor closed head injury after falling off a trampoline. She had no LOC and 2 episodes of emesis.	What is this child's risk of a TBI that needs neurosurgical intervention? What are the harms of a CT scan in terms of radiation, sedation, and costs?	PECARN study risk calculation shows intermediate (0.8%) TBI risk.[16]	Shared decision-making with family on options of observing for a few more hours in the ED for worsening symptoms versus risks of sedation and incidental findings on imaging.
Inpatient	A 6 y old initially admitted for peripheral IV antibiotics for acute hematogenous osteomyelitis is now afebrile, clinically improved, and has a significant decline in C-reactive protein.	By what route should additional antibiotics be administered? What are the costs of PICC lines (including placement, risk of clots, infection, mechanical complications) versus oral antibiotics (including concerns about compliance).	Large study showing equivalent cure rates for oral and IV antibiotics, but with higher risks for IV antibiotics administered at home via PICC after discharge.[17]	Shared decision-making with family; they opt for discharge on an oral agent with weekly follow-up.

AAN, American Academy of Neurology; AAP, American Academy of Pediatrics; CT, computed tomography; ED, emergency department; IV, intravenous; PECARN, Pediatric Emergency Care Applied Research Network; PICC, peripherally inserted central catheter; TBI, traumatic brain injury.

CONCLUSIONS

With almost half of excess health care costs related to decision-making at the clinician level, opportunities to teach the incorporation of high-value care at the level of the clinical encounter are plentiful. Clinical teachers can bend the health care cost curve downward by teaching and role modeling high-value care. The tools presented in this article can help clinical teachers structure lessons in high-value care in daily clinical encounters. Highlighting the underlying bioethical principles and giving thoughtful consideration of options while meeting the best interests of patients and families will assist in incorporating the concept of value in clinical reasoning and medical decision-making. Great clinical teachers are well positioned to demonstrate in both practice and teaching how "doing less" in appropriate situations is safe, family-centered, evidence-based, and ethical.

ACKNOWLEDGMENTS

We thank the other members of the Council on Medical Student Education in Pediatrics Curriculum Taskforce subcommittee on teaching high-value pediatrics for stimulating many of the ideas included in this article: Lauren Walker, MD, Marta King, MD, MEd, Starla Martinez, MD, Brian Good, MD, Rukmani Vasan, MD, and Jeanine Ronan, MD. We also thank Alan Schroeder, MD, Matthew Garber, MD, and Gautham Suresh, MD, MPH, for their thoughtful review of this manuscript.

ABBREVIATIONS

PPI: Prepare, Process, Initiate
SOAP-V: Subjective, Objective, Assessment, Plan, Value

REFERENCES

1. Welch HG, Schwartz LM, Woloshin S. *Overdiagnosed: Making People Sick in the Pursuit of Health.* Boston, MA: Beacon Press; 2011

2. Berwick DM, Hackbarth AD. Eliminating waste in US health care. *JAMA.* 2012;307(14):1513–1516

3. ABIM Foundation. Choosing Wisely physician and patient lists. Available at www.choosingwisely.org/doctor-patient-lists/. Accessed August 4, 2016

4. Moser EM, Huang GC, Packer CD, et al. SOAP-V: Introducing a method to empower medical students to be change agents in bending the cost curve. *J Hosp Med.* 2016;11(3):217–220

5. Moses H III, Matheson DH, Dorsey ER, George BP, Sadoff D, Yoshimura S. The anatomy of health care in the United States. *JAMA.* 2013;310(18):1947–1963

6. Himmelstein DU, Warren E, Thorne D, Woolhandler S. Illness and injury as contributors to bankruptcy. *Health*

Aff (Millwood). 2005;(Suppl Web Exclusives):W5-63–W5-73

7. Auerbach DI, Kellermann AL. A decade of health care cost growth has wiped out real income gains for an average US family. *Health Aff (Millwood)*. 2011;30(9):1630–1636

8. Schroeder AR, Harris SJ, Newman TB. Safely doing less: a missing component of the patient safety dialogue. *Pediatrics*. 2011;128(6). Available at: www.pediatrics.org/cgi/content/full/128/6/e1596

9. Coon ER, Quinonez RA, Moyer VA, Schroeder AR. Overdiagnosis: how our compulsion for diagnosis may be harming children. *Pediatrics*. 2014;134(5):1013–1023

10. Detsky AS, Verma AA. A new model for medical education: celebrating restraint. *JAMA*. 2012;308(13):1329–1330

11. Pellerin MA, Elwyn G, Rousseau M, Stacey D, Robitaille H, Légaré F. Toward shared decision making: using the OPTION scale to analyze resident-patient consultations in family medicine. *Acad Med*. 2011;86(8):1010–1018

12. Chung EY, Yardley J. Are there risks associated with empiric acid suppression treatment of infants and children suspected of having gastroesophageal reflux disease? *Hosp Pediatr*. 2013;3(1):16–23

13. Subcommittee on Febrile Seizures; American Academy of Pediatrics. Neurodiagnostic evaluation of the child with a simple febrile seizure. *Pediatrics*. 2011;127(2):389–394

14. American Academy of Pediatrics Subcommittee on Hyperbilirubinemia. Management of hyperbilirubinemia in the newborn infant 35 or more weeks of gestation. *Pediatrics*. 2004;114(1):297–316

15. Newman TB, Kuzniewicz MW, Liljestrand P, Wi S, McCulloch C, Escobar GJ. Numbers needed to treat with phototherapy according to American Academy of Pediatrics guidelines. *Pediatrics*. 2009;123(5):1352–1359

16. Kuppermann N, Holmes JF, Dayan PS, et al; Pediatric Emergency Care Applied Research Network (PECARN). Identification of children at very low risk of clinically-important brain injuries after head trauma: a prospective cohort study. *Lancet*. 2009;374(9696):1160–1170

17. Keren R, Shah SS, Srivastava R, et al; Pediatric Research in Inpatient Settings Network. Comparative effectiveness of intravenous vs oral antibiotics for postdischarge treatment of acute osteomyelitis in children. *JAMA Pediatr*. 2015;169(2):120–128

18. Ralston SL, Schroeder AR. Doing more vs doing good: aligning our ethical principles from the personal to the societal. *JAMA Pediatr*. 2015;169(12):1085–1086